# SUGAR DET

# BEGINNERS

Easy to Follow Recipes to Help Eliminate Sugar Cravings

(Energy Boosting Recipes and Tips on Staying Sugar Free)

**Robert Burke**

Published by Alex Howard

# © **Robert Burke**

*Sugar Detox for Beginners: Easy to Follow Recipes to Help Eliminate Sugar Cravings (Energy Boosting Recipes and Tips on Staying Sugar Free)*

**ISBN 978-1-990169-87-8**

**Legal & Disclaimer**

The information contained in this book is not designed to replace or take the place of any form of medicine or professional medical advice. The information in this book has been provided for educational and entertainment purposes only.

# Table of contents

Part 1 ............................................................................................ 1

Introduction ................................................................................ 2

Chapter 1: Sugar Detox .............................................................. 3

Chapter 2: Overcome Your Sugar Detox Symptoms .................. 9

Chapter 3: How To Overcome Sugar Addiction........................ 12

Chapter 4: Sugar Detox Preparation Checklist ....................... 16

Chapter 5: Allowed And Prohibited Food List ......................... 18

Chapter 6: Supplement Recommendations.............................. 25

Chapter 7: Dining Out During Your Sugar Detox ................... 27

Chapter 8: Frequently Asked Questions ................................. 29

Chapter 9: 10 Day Detox Plan ................................................. 35

Breakfast Recipes....................................................................... 36

Avocado Toasts With Fried Eggs And Garlic Shrimp............... 36

Almond Milk, Cinnamon Oatmeal ........................................... 38

Spinach And Mushroom Omelette............................................ 39

Bacon With Potato Hash And Egg Over Roasted Cauliflower 40

Charred Cauliflower With Almonds And Shishito Peppers.... 41

Mediterranean Breakfast Tostadas......................................... 42

Vanilla Chia Pudding ................................................................ 43

Blueberry Muffins...................................................................... 44

Veggie Quinoa Breakfast Bowl ................................................ 45

Buckwheat, Oat And Apple Muffins......................................... 45

Lunch Recipes............................................................................. 47

Crunchy Detox Salad ................................................................ 47

Pumpkin Lentil Soup................................................................. 48

Black Bean Lettuce Wraps With Cilantro Lime Rice And Grilled Corn Salsa................................................................49

Quinoa-Cranberry Grilled Chicken Salad ........................................50

Tomato And White Bean Salad With Homemade Pesto And Oven-Roasted Yellow Squash..........................................................51

Crockpot Black Bean, Sweet Potato, And Quinoa Chili............53

Slow Roasted Herb Roast Beef..........................................................54

Pan-Roasted Chicken Thighs With Charred Lemon, Sage, And Rosemary................................................................................................54

Beef Stir Fry With Onions And Peppers..........................................55

Pork Adobado........................................................................................56

Dinner Recipes......................................................................................57

Butternut Squash And Wild Rice Salad With Balsamic Dressing...................................................................................................57

Sweet Potato Kale Lentil Soup..........................................................59

Quinoa Salad And Lime Orange Dressing.......................................59

Vegan Chickpea, Cauliflower, And Potato Curry..........................61

Lemon Chicken Stew............................................................................62

Quinoa, Sweet Potato, And Black Bean Burger............................63

California Avocado, Veggie, Rice And Chicken Bowls.................66

Kale Soup ...............................................................................................68

Spaghetti Squash, Sausage And Kale Boats ..................................69

Greek Turkey Burgers .........................................................................70

Snacks.....................................................................................................71

Dill Crackers .........................................................................................71

Buttermilk Buns ...................................................................................72

Celery Root Cakes ...............................................................................73

Sundried Tomato Hummus.................................................................74

Smoky Lime Nut Mix ........................................................ 75

Kale Chips ..................................................................... 76

Turkey Jerky .................................................................. 77

Coconut Chia Seed Pudding ............................................. 77

Avocado With Poppy Seeds And Lemon .............................. 78

Juicy Green Booster ........................................................ 78

Chapter 10: Life Without Sugar ........................................ 80

Chapter 11: 10 Low Carb Ice Creams ................................. 82

1) Chocolate And Peanut Butter Ice Cream! ....................... 82

2) Chocolate Ice Cream ................................................... 83

3) Sugar Free Peanut Butter Ice Cream ............................. 85

4) Avocado Sorbet .......................................................... 86

5) Peanut Butter Sticks ................................................... 86

6) Coconut Ice Cream ...................................................... 87

7) Lemon Poppy Seed Ice Cream ....................................... 88

8) Mint Fudge Ice Cream .................................................. 89

9) Frozen Yoghurt Ice Cream ............................................ 91

10) Coffee Ice Cream ...................................................... 92

Chapter 12: 10 Low Carb Slushies .................................... 94

1) The Fruit Slushy ......................................................... 94

2) The Coke Slushy ......................................................... 95

3) Kool-Aid Slushy .......................................................... 95

4) The Organic Slushy ..................................................... 96

5) The Exotic Slushy ....................................................... 97

6) Chocolate Slushy ........................................................ 97

7) Peach Slushy .............................................................. 98

8) The Mango Slushy ....................................................... 99

9) Banana Slushy Surprise ........................................................99

Chapter 12:10 Low Carb Cocktails ....................................101

1) Standard Spirit & Mixer ..................................................101

2) Grape & Pineapple Fizz ..................................................101

3) Margarita..........................................................................102

4) Strawberry Vodka............................................................103

5) Vodka Melon....................................................................103

6) Spicy Bloody Mary ..........................................................104

7) Red Wine Surprise..........................................................105

8) The Mojito........................................................................106

9) Pina Colada......................................................................107

Conclusion............................................................................109

Part 2....................................................................................110

Introduction ........................................................................111

Chapter 1: An Overview Of The 21-Day Sugar Detox Diet: What It Is And How It Can Benefit You.........................113

Chapter 2: A Few Tips To Guide You Toward Success On The 21-Day Sugar Detox Diet ..............................................117

Chapter 3: Breakfast Recipes For The 21-Day Sugar Detox Diet........................................................................................120

Baked Cheesy Spinach Eggs ..............................................120

Sante-Fe Mini Frittatas.......................................................122

Breakfast Meatballs ............................................................124

Banana Pancakes.................................................................125

Chapter 4: Main Course Recipes For The 21-Day Sugar Detox Diet........................................................................................126

Lemon Garlic Chicken Drumsticks ....................................126

Meatloaf................................................................................128

Broccoli Mushroom Chicken Casserole.................................130

Garlic Dijon Salmon ..............................................................132

Chicken Cordon Bleu..............................................................133

Grilled Shrimp ........................................................................135

Garlic-Y Prime Rib..................................................................137

Chapter 5: Side Dish Recipes For The 21-Day Sugar Detox Diet 138

Fresh Zucchini Noodles..........................................................138

Cooked 'Zoodles'......................................................................139

Cheesy 'Bread' Sticks..............................................................140

Turkey 'Noodle' Soup..............................................................142

Smothered Green Beans..........................................................144

Prosciutto Wrapped Asparagus.............................................145

Creamy Cucumber Salad ........................................................146

Chapter 6: Snack And Dessert Recipes For The 21-Day Detox Diet..................................................................................147

Mini Zucchini Cheese Bites....................................................147

Spicy Mediterranean Dip........................................................149

Low-Carb Sushi........................................................................150

Pumpkin Custard ....................................................................151

Kale Chips.................................................................................152

Baked Cinnamon Apples Topped With Almonds ..................153

Pepperoni Pizza Bites..............................................................154

Sugar Busters Diet Recipes And Meal Plan...........................156

Easy And Delicious Breakfast Recipes..................................156

Avocado Coconut Green Smoothie .......................................156

Mixed Berry Coconut Smoothie ............................................157

Coconut Flour Waffles ................................................ 158

Blueberry Almond Pancakes ..................................... 159

Spinach And Tomato Omelette .................................. 161

Cucumber Salad With Fried Hemp Tofu ................... 162

Zucchini Breakfast Patties ........................................ 164

Healthy, Filling Lunch Recipes ................................. 166

Kale And Broccoli Egg White Quiche ........................ 166

Spinach And Mushroom Frittata .............................. 168

Baked Broccoli And Marinated Hemp Fu ................. 170

White Bean Soup With Kale And Wild Rice .............. 172

Broccoli And Fava Bean Salad .................................. 174

Grilled Vegetables And Hemp Tofu .......................... 176

Quinoa -Fava Green Salad With Avocado Sauce ....... 178

Vegetable Pasta Dinner Recipes .............................. 180

Carrot Noodles With Spicy Peanut Sauce ................ 180

Butternut Squash Noodles With Bean Bolognese ..... 182

Cucumber Noodles In Creamy Coconut Mushroom Sauce ... 184

Spinach Zucchini Lasagna With Caramelized Onions ........... 186

Conclusion ................................................................ 189

# Part 1

# Introduction

Do you feel sluggish and tired every day? Do you suffer from constant aches, pain and weight gain problems? Do you want to take back control of your health, body shape, and life? Then this book on sugar detox is for you.

Habitual consumption of high amounts of sugar leads to various health problems such as cardiovascular diseases, weight gain, diabetes, false craving, skin problems, and rapid aging. Various studies show that sugar is more addictive than cocaine, and today, most Americans are addicted to sugar-rich foods. Often, people fail to overcome sugar addiction with a regular diet. The reason is as they go through withdrawal, sugar craving makes it extremely difficult to stick to the diet. To overcome your sugar addiction, you need a detox plan. This guide is designed to help you effectively and quickly cut sugar from your diet without the withdrawal syndromes. The guide helps you to end your sugar cravings, increase your energy and lose weight naturally. The book includes the 10-day sugar detox plan. A Sugar detox plan can include both vegetarian and non-vegetarian recipes, and the book offers both types of recipes.

The detox plan will improve your mental and physical health and provide lasting energy. You will experience renewed energy, health and happiness from the real, whole, nutrient-rich foods that the detox plan offers. Whether you are suffering from diseases such as diabetes, high blood pressure, high cholesterol; facing a weight gain problem, or simply addicted to sugar and want to live a healthier life, this book on sugar detox can help you achieve the healthier version of you. This 10-day sugar detox is a whole-foods based diet plan that is easy to follow, effective and helps you quit sugar within weeks.

# Chapter 1: Sugar Detox

**The Truth About Sugar**

There are two types of sugar. The first is the natural sugar that is naturally present in foods such as fruits, grain, vegetables, and legumes. The second type of sugar is called the free sugars, also known as added sugars. Free sugars are added to beverages and food by the cook, manufacturer or the consumer. It also includes sugars naturally present in fruit juices; fruit juice concentrates, honey and syrups. Data provided by CDC (Centers for Disease Control and Prevention) shows that the average American adult gets about 13% of their daily calorie intake from processed and sugar rich foods. Men, on average, get an additional 335 calories daily from added sugar and women get about 239 added calories daily. This eating habit leads to food addiction, overeating, overweight, and blood sugar swings.

**Names of Sugar.**

Free sugar is called by many different names. The following are the 25 most common names for sugar:


- Sugar/ Sucrose
- High fructose corn syrup (HFCS)
- Agave Nectar
- Beet sugar
- Blackstrap molasses
- Cane juice crystals
- Cane sugar
- Caramel
- Castor sugar
- Coconut sugar

- Confectioner's sugar
- Date sugar
- Fruit juice
- Fruit juice concentrate
- Honey
- Icing sugar
- Maple syrup
- Molasses
- Raw sugar
- Refiner's sugar
- Brown rice syrup
- Corn syrup
- Glucose
- Rice syrup
- Fructose

**Spot the Hidden Sugar**

- Diet and low-fat foods are usually loaded with extra sugar to enhance their taste.
- Even savory foods, like ready-made sauces and soups, contain added sugar.
- On average, a can of soft drink contains about seven tsp. of sugar.
- New varieties of sweeter apples are cultivated to satisfy our desire for sweeter fruits.

Photo: fda.gov

Read the label

Here are a few tips for you to know how much sugar is in your food.

- On the nutrition panel, look at the carbs as sugars. This includes both natural and free sugars. More than 22.5g per 100g is high and less than 5g per 100g is low.
- Check the ingredients list for anything ending with ose (maltose, lactose, fructose, sucrose, glucose). All of these are different forms of sugars.
- Know the substitutes, for example, mannitol, sorbitol, xylitol. These sugars occur naturally in small amounts in fruits and plants and are added in low-calorie products to make the food sweet, but with fewer calories.

**Ways to Cut Down on Your Sugar**

Making a few adjustments to your diet can help cut down on your sugar consumption.

- Lower the sugar to your hot drinks such as tea or coffee. Do it gradually so your taste buds can adjust. Add cinnamon to your hot chocolate or cappuccino. It adds flavor without the sweetness.
- Avoid low-fat diet foods that are loaded with sugar. Eat smaller portions of foods regularly.
- Be wary of sugar-free foods. They often contain artificial sweeteners like aspartame, saccharin, and sucralose. These sweeteners lead to over-eating.
- Balance your carb intake with lean protein like turkey, chicken, and fish. Protein rich foods slow down food absorption and lower cravings.
- Avoid white bread, white rice and eat whole grain bread, brown rice, and pasta.
- Reduce the sugar in recipes and add spices to enhance the taste and flavor.
- Keep fruit juice, sweet soft drinks and alcohol consumption minimum. Enjoy herbal teas, or water flavored with citrus fruits.

- Eat sugar-rich foods such as muffins and cakes on special occasions only.
- Use fruit for sweetness instead of added sugar.

**Why Sugar is a Problem for You: Sugar and Your Health**

Just like morphine, heroin, and painkillers, sugar is also an addictive substance. Here is how sugar harms your health:

- Sugar causes irregular blood glucose levels: Unstable blood sugar leads to fatigue, mood swings, headaches and cravings for more sugar. When you eat sugar, you feel good, but after a few hours, the effects subdue, which results in more sugar craving and hunger.
- Sugar increases your risk of various diseases: Sugar increases your risk of obesity, heart disease, and diabetes. Many studies also show that sugar-rich diets can lead to different types of cancer.
- Sugar restricts immune function: Sugar interferes with immune function. When your immune function is affected, infections and diseases are more likely.
- Sugar rich diet results in chromium deficiency: If you follow a sugar-rich diet, your body won't have enough trace mineral chromium. Chromium's main job is to regulate blood sugar. According to published data, 90% Americans are suffering a chromium deficiency. Chromium is found a variety of plant foods, seafood, and animal foods.
- Sugar accelerates aging: In a process called glycation, sugar ages your body tissues, including your arteries, organs, and skin. The more sugar you consume, the quicker this aging process happens in your body.
- Sugar causes tooth decay: Aside from all the serious and life-threatening effects of sugar, sugar also causes basic damage such as tooth decay.

- Sugar can cause gum disease: Sugar can cause gum disease, and studies show that gum disease can lead to coronary artery disease.
- Sugar affects behavior and cognition in children: Millions of parents confirm that sugar-rich diet changes the behavior of their children (makes them more edgy and restless) and lowers their ability to remember things.
- Sugar increases stress: Eating sugar rich foods causes a blood-sugar spike. There is a compensatory dive which causes your body to release stress hormones such as cortisol, epinephrine, and adrenaline. These hormones raise blood sugar and give your body a quick energy boost. However, the problem is these hormones can make you shaky, irritable and anxious.
- Sugar replaces important nutrients: Data provided by the USDA shows that people who follow a sugar-rich diet have the lowest intake of important nutrients – especially iron, magnesium, phosphorous, calcium, folate, Vitamin A, B-12, and C.

**Sugar Detox Symptoms**

Once you limit or stop consuming sugar, your body can have quite a reaction. Here are some common symptoms of sugar withdrawal.

- Overeating
- You strongly feel the urge to nap
- Heavy naps during the middle of the day
- Intense thirst
- Frequent urination
- Intense hunger
- You are not satisfied even after eating enough
- Possible weight gain

- Constipation or diarrhea
- Gas
- Bloating
- Overspending on stuff
- Anticipated rituals unfulfilled
- Boredom
- Loss of sleep
- Lack of motivation
- Strange dreams
- Anxiousness
- Depression
- Crankiness
- Low energy
- Sweating (without any physical strain)
- Jitters/shaky hands

# Chapter 2: Overcome Your Sugar Detox Symptoms

In this chapter, we are going to discuss how you can overcome your sugar detox symptoms:

- Cutting back gradually and cold turkey method: If currently, you are following a high sugar diet, then cutting back gradually can be the best strategy for you. Gradually lower your sugar intake over a few days or a couple of weeks. For example, as a first step towards the sugar detox, you can stop drinking all sugar-sweetened beverages and then avoid all processed foods the subsequent week. If you gradually lower your sugar intake, you will suffer less from the side effects of sugar detox.

- Satisfy your cravings without eating sugar: Sugar craving is one of the most intense side effects of sugar withdrawal. Include healthier alternatives of sugar in your diet and subdue your sugar cravings. For examples, fruit contains healthy natural sugar and also contain fiber, antioxidants, vitamins, and minerals. Eating fruits placate your sugar craving, provide a multitude of health benefits and prevent a rapid spike in blood sugar. Grapes, oranges, strawberries, and apples all make excellent snacks and keeps your sugar craving under control.

- Stay active: If you often find yourself lingering around the kitchen looking for food, do something productive to distract yourself, such as exercising. Working out is an effective way to reduce stress, feel great and avoid symptoms like nausea and headaches. Exercise is also an excellent method for keeping anxiety, mood swings and depression induced by sugar withdrawal at bay.

- Keep blood sugar regular: Some people report experiences of tremors or feeling shaky after they cut off sugar. These symptoms are linked to low blood sugar and can be avoided easily. If you do start getting the shakes, eat regularly and incorporate more small snacks into your diet. Choose protein-rich foods; they absorb slowly and keep you feeling full and satisfied for longer. Eating protein also helps stabilize blood sugars.

- Have an Epsom salt bath: Pains, aches and flu-like symptoms are all linked with symptoms of sugar detox. An Epson salt bath is one of the best ways to relieve muscle pains. This also helps irritation, soreness, cramps, and inflammation in muscles and joints caused by sugar detox. To prepare the bath, add 1 or 2 cups of Epsom salt to your bath and soak for about 20 minutes to get the best results. Also, you can use an Epsom salt compress to relieve more localized pains and aches.

- Focus on healthy choices: Before you start sugar detox, remove all tempting sugar rich foods from your house and replace them with healthy ones. Eat fruits and veggies as snacks. Prepare a snack box supplied with apple slices, carrots, celery sticks, hard-boiled eggs, nuts and other healthy favorites.

- Stay hydrated: Most of us don't drink enough water. Often when you are feeling thirsty, you start to crave for sweets. The next time you crave for a sugar rich food, drink a glass of water and wait 10 minutes to see how you feel. Aim for eight 8 oz. glasses of water daily to stay hydrated. If you exercise regularly, then increase your water intake.

- De-stress: Sugar withdrawals can cause symptoms like mood swings, anxiety, and depression. Minimizing your stress can make the process of quitting sugar easier. Practicing meditation and yoga are both great ways to lower your stress and relax. Taking a break from computer screens and technology for part of the day is also helpful.

- Get enough sleep: Getting enough sleep can make your sugar detox plan run smoother. When you sleep less, you crave more sugar and carb-rich foods and make your sugar detox plan harder to follow. When you start to cut back on sugar, your sleep is disrupted, and you feel tired because you are not getting the energy spike from eating sugar. Sleep 7 to 8 hours every night so your body can rest and fully recover. Some better sleep habits include: going to bed at the same time every day even on weekends, keeping your bedroom cool, minimizing sound, and reading or listening to soft music before sleep.

# Chapter 3: How To Overcome Sugar Addiction

Let's discuss how you can overcome your sugar addiction. Here are some great tips and strategies you can follow to overcome your sugar addiction.

- Get the sweet stuff out of the house: Remove all sugar and processed foods from your house. You can drastically increase your ability to resist the temptation of sugar-rich foods by removing all processed and sugar rich foods. Look through your pantry, kitchen and cupboards for bread, baked goods, fat-free yogurts, snack bars, cereals, and all sugary drinks. Remove them from your house and stay committed not to bring these foods back into your home until you overcome your sugar addiction.

- Eat a balanced breakfast: Often, your body craves for sugar because your body hasn't received the nutrients it really craves. Eating a well-rounded breakfast is the easiest way to minimize or eliminate these deficiencies.

- Eat more real food: Eat real foods. This means eating foods with substance, such as nut butter, cheese, avocado, Greek yogurt, beans, eggs, fish, and meat. When you are addicted to sugar, you tend to eat more carb and sugar rich foods and not enough healthy fats and protein. This means you are not fully satisfied and always go for the sweet stuff.

- Substitute whole fruit for sweets: Fruit contains fructose, which metabolizes differently from sugar-rich foods. Eating fruits subdues your sugar addiction and satisfies your need for a treat. Also, be careful when eating cherries or grapes because they are high in sugar.

- Ditch artificial sweeteners: Large amounts of these can make you desire sweet food, so ditch saccharine, sucralose, and aspartame.
- Manage your magnesium levels: Studies show that people crave for sugar-rich treats such as chocolate because they are magnesium deficient. Eat magnesium-rich dark leafy greens, nuts, legumes, almonds, pumpkin seeds, and tofu to boost your magnesium levels.
- If you feel hungry, eat a meal: Understand that craving is not same as hunger. Craving is not your body calling for energy. It is your brain calling for something that releases a lot of dopamine. However, if you are hungry and craving for sugar, then you make the situation much worse. A hunger paired with a craving is a powerful drive that most people have a hard time overcoming. If you are hungry and get a craving, then eat some real food. Eating real food instead of food that you crave (such as ice cream) may not feel very appetizing, but do it anyway.
- Take a hot shower: A lot of people found this technique very helpful. When you crave sugar rich foods, take a hot shower for at least 5 to 10 minutes. Once you have finished your hot shower, your craving will most likely be gone.
- Prepare healthy snacks in bulk: Prepare healthy snacks in batches and carry some with you all the time. Often, sugar addiction is difficult because snacks that people eat are mostly loaded with refined grains and sugar. Granola bars, yogurt, crackers, snack bars, cookies and many other common snack items will prolong your sugar addiction. Find a few healthy snacks that are free from highly processed ingredients and sugar and prepare a large batch every few days. Store and take them with you anywhere you go.
- The coffee experiment: If you are addicted to sugar, then you take a lot of sugar (like 5 packets) with your coffee. So, first, subtract one. Your coffee may not taste as great at first,

but continue the process and after 2 weeks, bring the number of sugar packets to only one and then none. The key is to cut back gradually.

- Reduce your dessert-eating frequency: If you have developed a habit of eating cakes after dinner every other day, then reduce to two days a week, then one day and over time eat cakes only on special occasions. Also, choose your desserts wisely. For example, fresh fruit with a dollop of whipped cream is a good choice.

- Drink plenty of water: Often you may think that your body is asking for sugar, but actually, it is dehydrated and craving water. Whenever you have a sugar craving, drink water. In 8 oz. water, add 5 drops of Stevia and juice of a ½ lemon for a healthy lemonade. Also, you can try a warm cup of green tea with stevia. Green drinks are loaded with nutrition, boost your energy and lower your craving for processed foods and sugar.

- Eat more sea vegetables: Seaweed and sea vegetables are rich in vitamins and minerals and make a healthy snack. Anything with sugar depletes minerals from your body. On the other hand, sea vegetables also have a high mineral content. Include sea vegetables in your meals.

- Enjoy fermented foods and drinks: Studies show that consuming fermented foods and drinks are one of the effective ways to reduce or even eliminate cravings for sugar. Here are some fermented foods: pickles, tempeh, kimchi, sauerkraut, kombucha, kefir, natto, and yogurt.

- Say no to fat-free products: Say no to fat-free products because they are fat-free, but not sugar-free. For examples, fat-free salad dressing, fat-free cookies or cakes, fat-free muffins, puddings, and reduced-fat peanut butter.

- Meditate and manage your stress: If you are living a stressful life, then you will have difficulty beating your sugar craving. Meditation can help you subdue your sugar craving by lowering stress. Prolonged stress boosts the production of the stress hormone cortisol, which increases your blood sugar level. This creates a vicious cycle that creates sugar cravings and damages your adrenals. Practicing a short meditation before meals can help you relax during your mealtime. When you are relaxed during mealtime, your body digests foods and absorbs nutrients better.

- Get better quality sleep every night: Studies show that your sugar addiction will intensify if you are not getting enough quality sleep at night.

- Have a backup plan: If your sugar craving is just uncontrollable, then have backup plans to overcome it. For example, listen to some music, go for a walk, eat a piece of fruit, read a fun article, call or text a friend. Distractions will help you overcome your sugar addiction. From the examples, going for a walk is a highly effective strategy, and it is even better if you can run. Walking helps you in two ways; first, you are distancing yourself from sugar-rich foods that you are eager to eat. Second, walking or running will release endorphins, which help turn the craving off. If it is not possible for you to go outside, do a few body weight squats, push-ups, burpees, or any other body weight exercise.

# Chapter 4: Sugar Detox Preparation Checklist

It is important that you prepare yourself for the sugar detox plan. Here is the checklist:

- Understand what really goes on in your body when you are addicted to sugar. This first part of the book will help you a great deal. Also, read other books on the topic.
- You are starting as a beginner. So you have to follow all the necessary steps exactly.
- Review the Yes/No list of foods.
- When you are on the sugar detox, you can't eat certain foods. So make a list of foods that you need to replace.
- You are following a meal plan. So print a "yes" food list and follow it when shopping.
- Shop for any pantry items you need.
- If for any reason, you are unable to buy food items locally, shop online.
- Check your fridge and pantry for off-plan ingredients and foods. Either donate them, finish eating them before your detox plan begins, toss them in the trash or set them aside while you are on the plan.
- Find a friend and/or family member to join you.
- Get your supplements online or from your local food store.
- Join various online and social media forums that are focused on sugar detox plan.
- If you have to make slow cooker or soup recipes for your detox plan, make no sugar added broths and freeze them, so they are ready when you need them.

16

- Carry healthy snacks with (such as jerky, nuts, nut butter) you, so you can have a detox friendly snack whenever you need it.
- Check and check your pantry and fridge again to make sure you eliminated all the off-plan items. If you are living with someone who is not following the plan, create separate shelves in the pantry and fridge so the items don't get mixed up.
- Before you start day 1, have meals planned and/or cooked and ready to go. Preparation is your biggest key to success. Success in day 1 will help you go along with the detox plan.

# Chapter 5: Allowed And Prohibited Food List

In this chapter, we are going to discuss a "yes" and "no" food list that you have to follow while you are on sugar detox plan

**"Yes" Food List**

Meat, fish, and eggs


- Eggs
- All seafood
- All meats, including cured and deli meats like prosciutto, pancetta, bacon, etc.

Vegetables

Fruit
1 fruit daily is allowed

- Bananas, green-tipped/not quite ripe
- Grapefruit
- Green/Granny Smith apples
- Lime
- Lemon

Nuts/Seeds (whole, flour or butter)

Fats and Oils


- Sesame oil
- Olives, olive oil
- Flax oil

- Coconut oil
- Avocados, avocado oil
- Butter, ghee, classified butter
- Animal fats

Dairy (only full-fat)

- Kefir, plain
- Sour cream
- Heavy cream
- Half & half
- Milk, whole only
- Cheese, cream cheese, cottage cheese

Beverages

- Water
- Teas: black, white, green, herbal, etc. unsweetened
- Seltzer, club soda
- Mineral water
- Coffee, espresso
- Coconut milk, coconut cream, full-fat
- Almond milk, homemade/unsweetened

Condiments/Misc.

- Vinegar: balsamic, apple cider, rice, distilled, red wine, sherry, white
- Spices & herbs: all are acceptable. Check pre-mixed blends for hidden sugar content

- Salad dressings, homemade
- Nutritional/Brewer's yeast
- Mustard, gluten-free verities
- Healthy homemade mayonnaise
- Hummus made from cauliflower
- Extracts: almond, vanilla, vanilla bean, etc
- Sweetener-free ketchup
- Coconut aminos
- Broth, homemade only

Supplements

- 100% pure, protein powder with no other ingredients (100% egg white, whey, or hemp)
- Pure vitamin or mineral supplements
- Fermented cod liver oil, with or without flavor

**Limit Foods**

"Yes" foods with protein size limits

Vegetables and Starches (1 cup serving daily is allowed)

- Winter squash (assorted)
- Pumpkin
- Green peas
- Butternut squash
- Beets
- oAcorn squash

Grains/Legumes (1/2 cup serving daily is allowed - whole forms only – no flours)

- Sorghum
- Rice (wild, brown, white)
- Quinoa
- Millet
- Lentils
- Buckwheat
- Beans: red, pinto, navy garbanzo (chickpeas), fava, black
- Arrowroot
- Amaranth

Beverages (1 cup total daily is allowed)

- Kombucha, homebrewed or store-bought
- Coconut juice, coconut water (no added sweeteners)

## "No" Foods

Don't eat these foods while you are on sugar detox plan

Refined Carbohydrates

Vegetables & Starches

- Taro
- Tapioca, wheat & flour
- Sweet potatoes/yams
- Soybeans/edamame
- Plantains
- Corn, polenta, grits
- Cassava

Fruits (review the Yes and Limit foods lists for included fruits)

- Fresh & dried

Grains/Legumes

- Flours made from grains or beans (lentils, chickpeas, etc.)
- Wheat
- Spelt
- Soybeans/Edamame(including soy sauce, tofu, tempeh, natto, miso)
- Rye
- Kamut
- Barley

Nuts/Nut Butters

- Peanut
- Cashew

Sweeteners of any kind

- Completely avoid sweeteners
- Avoid anything sugar-free, diet or artificially sweetened (also, no gum)

Supplements

- Supplements that contain wheat, corn or soy

- Anything that includes sugar alcohols (xylitol, for example), sugar, sweeteners
- Shakeology and other similar blends

Beverages

- Protein powders that have more than one ingredient
- Sweet-tasting drinks (besides herbal teas)
- Soda (diet and regular)
- Milk: nonfat, skim, 1%, 2%, soy/rice/oat
- Juice
- Coffee drinks or shakes presweetened
- All alcohol

Condiments/Misc.

- Soy sauce, tamari
- Salad dressings, pre-made/store-bought
- Mayonnaise, store-brought
- Ketchup, store-bought
- Hummus made from garbanzo beans
- Broth/stock in a box/can

**Additional notes for those who need more carbohydrates**

Here are some modifications that may be right for you if:

- Work at a physically demanding job or live a very active lifestyle.
- Exercise regularly or participate in a high-intensity physical activity (for example, aerobic/cardio activity, endurance

athletics, CrossFit-style workouts, and interval training for more than 20 minutes at a time.

- Are pregnant or nursing

If you need more carbs, you could eat foods like sweet potatoes and potatoes, included a few recipes that include these items.

Recommended carbs per day

- Moderately active: 75 to 150 grams
- Highly active: 100 to 200+ grams
- Pregnant + nursing: 100+ grams

# Chapter 6: Supplement Recommendations

Once you start sugar detox, your body will crave sugar. Here are some natural, food-based approaches to curbing your sugar craving. Try these before you look to herbal or vitamin and mineral supplements for support. First, two natural drinks:

- Lemon water: Add a few drops of lemon juice or any other citrus fruit juice. Occasionally, you can add L-glutamine to it. They will help curb your sugar addiction.
- Herbal teas: You can add full-fat coconut milk to it. There are many varieties you can try such as licorice root tea, ginger, and peppermint. When drinking tea, use one tea bag several times instead of drinking very potent tea all day long.

Besides the above, you can try a few different herbs and supplements to lower your sugar craving. Start with a low dosage and increase dosage as you get used to it.

- Cinnamon: Cinnamon is an aromatic spice. Cinnamon helps to lower your sugar craving and also regulates blood sugar. Add cinnamon to your food or your tea and coffee according to taste. You can add cinnamon to lamb, beef and pork chops.
- L-Glutamine: It is an amino acid. Dietary sources of L-glutamine include high-protein foods like eggs, fish, chicken and beef. L-glutamine boosts metabolism, lowers sugar cravings, supports the repair of small intestines and improves gut function. If you are taking it in powder form, add 4 grams in water up to twice daily between meals.
- Magnesium: Magnesium is a mineral. Dietary sources include bone broth, dried herbs, scallops, halibut, oysters, salmon,

Swiss chard, broccoli, spinach, sunflower seeds and pumpkin seeds. Your body needs magnesium for over 300 enzymatic processes in the body. You can take 300 to 600 mg of magnesium malate or magnesium gluconate daily in capsule form. Or you can add 300 to 600 mg in your drink. Start with ½ tsp. and go up from there. You can take magnesium any time of the day, but after dinner is ideal.

- Chromium: Chromium is a mineral that can be found on shelves as Chelavite, Polynicotinate, and Chromium Picolinate. Dietary sources include dulse, kelp, dried seaweed paper, green apples with peel, peppers, liver, ripe tomatoes, romaine lettuce, onions, and eggs. Chromium helps increase insulin sensitivity, which has an effect on how well your body regulates blood sugar. Take 200 micrograms three times daily (total of 200 to 600 micrograms) with each meal.

- B Vitamins: B vitamin is a water-soluble vitamin. Dietary sources include meats, eggs, leafy greens, organic full-fat dairy, and liver. B Vitamins help combat fatigue. Take 100 milligrams twice a day for breakfast and lunch.

- Gymnema: It is a herb that is known as Gymnema Sylvestre. You can find it as liquid, powder, tablet, or capsule form. You can add the leaves of the herb in your tea. When placed in the mouth, it reduces the taste of the sugar and lowers your sugar cravings. Follow the instructions on the package. Take when you experience sugar craving.

# Chapter 7: Dining Out During Your Sugar Detox

You can follow your detox plan when you are cooking at home. However, when eating at restaurants, it is a different story. When you are dining out, it is difficult to avoid processed ingredients and hidden sugars. Here are some tips to help you enjoy restaurant food and stick with the sugar detox plan.

- Do some research and pick the restaurant yourself: Do some Google search and filter your search with words like Paleo, organic, farm to table and gluten free. These restaurants will be more accommodating to your detox needs. If necessary, call ahead to make sure they offer a flexible menu.
- Ask about ingredients: This step might seem intimidating and uncomfortable at first, but as you do it often, it will get easier. Ask if there are any hidden ingredients like flour, soy sauce, cheese or breadcrumbs. If the waiter is not sure, then make sure they go back and ask the chef. If the chef can come to talk to you, then it is even better. If the restaurant has a gluten free menu or gluten free option, then half the walk is already done for you.
- Focus on salads: Almost every restaurant serves some type of salad. Make sure to let them know to leave out croutons, cheese, sugar-rich dressings or any other ingredients that don't go with your detox plan. Avoid breaded or fried foods and choose proteins that are grilled. If the restaurant offers a build-your-own option, take advantage of that.
- Bring your own condiments: Sauces and dressing are often the culprits. Bring your own and avoid gluten, artificial sweeteners, and other sugar added ingredients.

- Hold the rice and the bun: Let the waiter know beforehand that you don't want certain items that usually comes with the dish. When ordering meals, be sure to say you don't want rice, bread, buns and bread baskets. Ordering bun-less sandwiches and burgers are a great option for you.
- Ask for substitutions: Ask for substitutions, for example, when getting a burger, ask for a salad or grilled or roasted veggies as a side instead of fries. If you are hesitant to bring your own dressing, ask the waiter if they provide vinegar and olive oil instead. Fresh lemon is also a great choice to season your salads and meat. If the restaurant uses vegetable oil to cook food ask them to use butter or olive oil instead. Also, if you ask them to hold the rice on a dish, substitute it with extra veggies.

Here are some more tips when dining out in certain restaurants:

- Mexican: Stay away from the heavy stuff, such as churros, stuffed tacos, and burritos. You can have one corn tortilla. Order lots of sautéed veggies, beans, guacamole, and proteins.
- Thai: Order veggies with proteins and go for seaweed salad and sashimi. Avoid any food items that are made with sugar, bad oil or MSG.
- All American restaurants: Totally avoid breaded/fried foods. Choose lettuce wrapped sandwiches and burgers. Ask for Dijon over ketchup and honey mustard. For salad dressing use fresh lemon juice and olive oil.

# Chapter 8: Frequently Asked Questions

**Now we are going to discuss frequently asked questions about sugar detox:**

- How is this detox program different from other detox, cleanse programs and nutrition challenges out there?

Many other programs help you eat better, lose weight and get healthier. However, this sugar detox program does all of that plus helps you diminish your sugar and carb cravings. Once you have given up sugar and sugar rich foods, natural foods will taste very sweet, and you will enjoy eating than ever before. From the "yes" list, you can see you are allowed to eat a lot of foods. At first, you may feel a bit overwhelmed, but it will get easier as the days pass.

- Can I create a sugar detox program on my own and follow it without needing this one?

The answer is yes and no. By simply removing sugar from your diet, you can start a sugar detox program, but removing sugar is only a part of the program. Remember only removing sugar doesn't always eliminate your craving. Subduing your craving and successfully avoiding the temptation of sugar-rich foods is also important. The program gives you a complete picture.

- Is the program a zero-sugar, zero-carb or low-carb program?

Not really. The detox program is all about processed foods, sugars and sweeteners. Also, the program includes real food carbohydrate sources and some natural sugars from whole foods. The amount of carb rich and natural sugar containing foods you can eat will be based on your activity levels and specific needs.

- Can I follow or try the program several times?

Yes, you can! Often many people try the program once every six or three months.

- What if I am pregnant or breastfeeding?

Some detox programs are not recommended for women who are pregnant or breastfeeding. However, this detox program is based on whole, real, natural foods. This is why many pregnant and breastfeeding women find this program very beneficial. The program is healthy for everyone, pregnant, breastfeeding or completely normal. If you are breastfeeding, you can add foods such as sweet potatoes, which make you, energized and support a healthy milk supply.

- Can I follow the detox plan permanently?

Yes, you can. Eating real, whole foods are always safe and healthy. The detox plan is a low-sugar, low-trigger-food diet and you can safely follow this program for life. The detox program is not a diet; it is a lifestyle. If you are following the program for life, you can do a few things to make it easier:

- Eat a square or two of organic 85% dark chocolate.
- Add a serving or two of seasonal fruits daily.
- Add more good carbs like plantains and sweet potatoes.
- Follow a similar diet plan such as grain-free diet, Paleo or whole-30 diet.
- Is there anyone who shouldn't follow the detox plan?

If you are living a very active lifestyle, a CrossFiter or an athlete, then wait until your event or training is completed.

- Does the detox program act as an anti-Candida diet?

You should not consider this detox program as a substitute for a professional treatment. If you are experiencing symptoms of Candida, then consult a healthcare practitioner to find the right plan for you.

- Can I modify the program to suit my own needs?

Follow the program faithfully, and only make any changes if you feel the need for it. The plan is about eating whole, real foods, so if you find another alternative which is better you can follow it.

**Questions Related to Food**

- Why are some fruits included in the diet while others aren't allowed?

The goal of the detox plan is to change your palate and your food habits. The detox plan will take you out of your sugar-rich comfort zone and introduce and allow only bland, sour, and fairly bitter fruits (such as grapefruit and under-ripe bananas) These fruits don't tend to taste very sweet or trigger sugar craving.

- Why are some nuts are included, and some excluded?

While other nuts are allowed, peanuts and cashews belong to "no" list. As mentioned earlier, the goal of the sugar detox plan is to change your palate and habits. Cashews trigger sweet-taste habits, and peanuts are known for the toxin load issue. This is why both of them are out.

- What can I drink besides water?

Besides water, lemon water, and herbal tea, you can enjoy coffee, black tea, white tea and green tea.

- What sauces and dressing can I use?

Only sugar-free sauces and dressings are allowed. So, it is best to use a homemade version or buy sugar-free options.

- Can I eat cured meat and bacon while on the detox plan?

Yes, you can eat bacon. Sugar is used in the curing process, but sugar isn't actually left in the resulting bacon. However, you have to avoid preservatives like sodium ascorbate, sodium phosphates, BHT, BHA and any other artificial ingredients.

- Why should I avoid FODMaps?

FODMaps are types of carbohydrates that can be difficult for people to digest. If you have any intolerances to FODMaps, it is better to avoid it.

- Should I avoid nightshades?

Nightshades contain specific alkaloid compounds that can be problematic for people who are suffering from inflammation and joint pain. Eggplant, peppers (bell and hot), white potatoes and tomatoes are most commonly consumed nightshades. People who are sensitive to nightshades should avoid these.

- Will I lose weight on the detox plan?

It is recommended that you don't weigh yourself while you are on the detox plan. Weigh yourself before you start and then once you have finished it. Avoiding sugar rich foods and processed foods and eating mainly whole, real foods often results in weight loss.

- I have noticed some changes to my digestion. Is it normal and what can I do?

If you are facing constipation problems while on the detox plan, it is highly recommended that you add some formatted foods like fermented pickles, kombucha (up to 8 ounces per day), raw sauerkraut. Also, add more soluble fiber into your diet if you are constipated. Butternut squash, parsnips, and carrots add soluble fiber to your diet. If you find that your eliminations are more frequent or looser than usual while on the detox plan, adding a cup of bone broth or supplementing with L-glutamine can be really helpful. If your digestion seems to be irritated and move more quickly than normal, then avoid nuts, seeds, and leafy greens, like collards and kale.

## Mindset and Habits

- Does following a detox plan show weakness? Why is my willpower not enough to overcome cravings?

Instead of a detox plan, some people think that self-control is enough to overcome sugar craving. However, the problem is our instincts tend to push us in a different direction. If there is sweet food readily available nearby, our instinct is to eat it. With a detox plan, you complexly remove sugar rich and processed foods and avoiding sugar becomes much easier.

- What should you do after the detox plan?

You may be thinking you have avoided foods that you like for a few days so now it is time to start eating them. But before you start to eat a piece of pizza, some cookies, a pile of candy or a glass of fruit juice, let's discuss some things:

- Before the detox plan, you tend to eat foods that make you spiral into eating more and more sugar-rich foods.
- After the detox plan, ask yourself how you feel now after you have lowered the amount of sugar and bad carb rich foods.
- Have you noticed a difference in your sleep quality? What about your digestive function? Must you have noticed improvement?
- Do you think going back to eating sugar, bad carbs, and processed foods will make you feel better or worse?
- So, you followed the sugar detox plan. Has the plan added more stress in your life or has it made it stress-free?
- After the detox plan, you need to reintroduce foods slowly.

## The Reintroducing Food Plan:

- The day after your detox plan, choose your favorite food to eat again.
- Reintroduce only one potentially problematic food at a time.
- Then, avoid eating that food again for the next two days.
- Notice any changes in the next 3 days after eating the food: digestive function (like diarrhea, loose stool, gas, bloating), appetite, energy, mood, headaches, inflammation and mental clarity.
- Your notes will be the best guides to whether you are sensitive to the food you just reintroduced. You have to observe up to 72 hours to notice any food sensitivity.
- Avoid reintroducing gluten-containing grains like spelt, rye, barley, and wheat.
- Next, think about how often you need to consume carb and sugar rich foods. Then, gradually reintroduce them one by one.

The next chapter includes sugar detox recipes. Remember, sugar detox recipes are meant to lower or eliminate sugar from your diet, and they can be both vegetarian and non-vegetarian recipes.

# Chapter 9: 10 Day Detox Plan

**10 Day Detox Plan**

### Day 1

Breakfast: Avocado Toasts with Fried Eggs and Garlic Shrimp
Lunch: Crunchy Detox Salad
Dinner: Butternut Squash and Wild Rice Salad with Balsamic Dressing

### Day 2

Breakfast: Almond Milk, Cinnamon Oatmeal
Lunch: Pumpkin Lentil Soup
Dinner: Sweet Potato Kale Lentil Soup

### Day 3

Breakfast: Spinach and Mushroom Omelette
Lunch: Black Bean Lettuce Wraps with Cilantro Lime Rice and Grilled Corn Salsa
Dinner: Quinoa Salad and Lime Orange Dressing

### Day 4

Breakfast: Bacon with Potato Hash and Egg Over Roasted Cauliflower
Lunch: Quinoa-Cranberry Grilled Chicken Salad
Dinner: Vegan Chickpea, Cauliflower, and Potato Curry

### Day 5

Breakfast: Charred Cauliflower with Almonds and Shishito Peppers
Lunch: Tomato and White Bean Salad with Homemade Pesto and Oven-Roasted Yellow Squash
Dinner: Lemon Chicken Stew

### Day 6

Breakfast: Mediterranean Breakfast Tostadas
Lunch: Crockpot Black Bean, Sweet Potato, and Quinoa Chili
Dinner: Quinoa, Sweet Potato, and Black Bean Burger

### Day 7

Breakfast: Vanilla Chia Pudding
Lunch: Slow Roasted Herb Roast Beef
Dinner: California Avocado, Veggie, Rice and Chicken Bowls

### Day 8

Breakfast: Blueberry Muffins
Lunch: Pan-Roasted Chicken Thighs with Charred Lemon, Sage, and Rosemary
Dinner: Kale Soup

### Day 9

Breakfast: Veggie Quinoa Breakfast Bowl
Lunch: Beef Stir Fry with Onions and Peppers
Dinner: Spaghetti Squash, Sausage, and Kale Boats

### Day 10

Breakfast: Buckwheat, Oat and Apple Muffins
Lunch: Pork Adobado
Dinner: Greek Turkey Burgers

# Breakfast Recipes

## Avocado Toasts With Fried Eggs And Garlic Shrimp

Ingredients for 2 servings

- Ripe avocado – 1 (cut in half lengthwise, pit removed and discarded)
- Fresh lemon juice – 1 ½ tsp.
- Cocktail tomatoes – 3, halved
- Freshly ground pepper
- Kosher salt
- Large eggs – 2
- Rustic bread – 2 slices
- Grated Parmesan cheese for serving

For the garlic shrimp

- Olive oil – 1 tbsp.
- Uncooked wild shrimp – ½ pound, peeled and deveined
- Garlic – 2 cloves, minced
- Lemon - ½ juiced
- Finely chopped parsley – 1 tsp.

Method

- Scoop the avocado from its skin and place in a small bowl. Add ¼ tsp. crushed red pepper flakes, 1 ½ tsp. lemon juice and mash the avocado. Season with salt to taste. To keep it from browning, press plastic wrap onto the surface of the avocado. Set aside.
- With a little olive oil, brush the cut side of the tomatoes and season with salt and pepper. Heat a medium skillet over medium-high heat. Add the tomatoes cut side down and allow to cook undisturbed until charred, about 4 to 5 minutes. Remove from the pan and cover with foil to keep warm.

- With a paper towel, pat shrimp dry and season with salt and pepper. In a large saucepan, heat 1 tbsp. of olive oil. Add the shrimp to the hot pan and cook for 2 minutes. Then add the garlic, flip the shrimp and cook until the shrimp had turned opaque and pink, about 2 minutes more. Careful not to burn the garlic.

- Remove the shrimp from the pan and place in a bowl. On the same pan, add the lemon juice, cook 15 seconds and scrape up any browned bits and garlic from the bottom of the pan. Add the pan juice to the shrimp, add chopped parsley and toss to coat.

- Heat a medium pan over medium heat. Add a little butter or olive oil and cook the egg in the hot pan until the yolks are still runny and whites are just set about 3 minutes.

- Meanwhile, brush the bread with a little olive oil and grill for 1 or 2 minutes on each side.

- To assemble: on each piece of toast, spread half of the avocado mixture in an even layer. Top each piece with half of the garlic shrimp and 3 charred tomatoes. Top with fried eggs and sprinkle with grated Parmesan.

- Serve.

# Almond Milk, Cinnamon Oatmeal

Ingredients for 8 servings (Cook time: 31 to 45 minutes)

- Water – 6 cups
- Homemade almond milk – 2 cups
- Organic coconut oil – 2 tbsp.
- Steel-cut oats – 2 cups
- Maldon sea salt – 1/8 tsp.
- Cinnamon – 1 tsp.

- Freshly ground nutmeg – ¼ tsp.
- Banana – 1, sliced
- Fresh blueberries – ¼ cup
- Chopped walnuts

Method

- Combine the milk and water in a large heavy-bottom saucepan. Over medium heat, bring the mixture to a simmer. In a large non-stick skillet, melt the coconut oil over medium heat. Once it starts to shine, add the oats and cook until the oats start to turn a bit golden, for about 2 minutes, stirring frequently.
- Add the oats to the water-milk mixture. Lower heat to medium-low and simmer for 20 minutes. Stir occasionally. Once the mixture starts to thicken, season with salt. Over low heat, let the oatmeal simmer for 12 to 15 minutes more. The mixture should become creamy.
- Remove the oatmeal from heat and set aside for 5 minutes to cool slightly.
- Add to the bowls and top with the toppings.

## Spinach And Mushroom Omelette

Ingredients for 2 servings (Cook time 11 to 15 minutes)

- Eggs – 4
- Extra virgin olive oil – 2 tbsp.
- Sea salt and ground pepper to taste
- Spinach leaves – 1 cup, roughly chopped
- Cremini Mushrooms – 1 cup, sliced

Method

- Whisk together milk, eggs, salt and pepper in a bowl.
- In a medium, non-stick skillet, add the olive oil and sauté mushrooms and spinach until fragrant. Drain and set aside.
- Add half of the egg mixture to the skillet. Once it starts to get firm, add half the mushroom and spinach mixture. Fold and repeat for the second egg.

# Bacon With Potato Hash And Egg Over Roasted Cauliflower

Ingredients for 2 servings (Cook time 5 to 10 minutes)

- Cauliflower – 1 head, cut into florets
- Bok choy – 1 head, cut and quartered
- Small red onion – 1, sliced
- Bacon – 2 to 3 strips, sautéed and cut
- Parsley – 3 tbsp. finely chopped
- Extra virgin olive oil – 1 tbsp.
- Russet or Yukon Gold potato – 1 medium, shredded
- Sea salt – ¼ tsp.
- Ground pepper – ¼ tsp.
- Eggs – 2, pastured

Method

- Place a pan over medium heat and add the strips. Sauté until crispy, about 30 seconds on each side. On a paper towel lined plate, place the bacon and set aside. Sauté the red onion for 3 to 5 minutes in the same pan. Add the cauliflower florets to the mix and sauté for 7 minutes or until lightly browned around the edges.

- Add the bok choy in the pan. Cover and lower heat to low. Caramelize the cauliflower for 12 minutes.
- Toss and set aside.
- For potato hash: in a new pan, place olive oil and cook shredded potatoes for 3 minutes. Add your favorite spices and season with salt and pepper. Cook for 1 or 2 minutes more. Don't allow the potatoes to get stuck in the bottom of the pan. Cover and cook for a few more minutes.
- Remove the hash brown and plate.
- For the egg: add bacon grease or leftover olive oil in the pan and add the eggs. Cover the eggs until it reaches your desired consistency, about 3 minutes.
- Place over cauliflower or potato hash.
- Serve.

# Charred Cauliflower With Almonds And Shishito Peppers

Ingredients for 2 servings (Cook time 16 to 30 minutes)

- Cauliflower – 1 head, trimmed, halved and cut into 1 ½ wedges
- Olive oil – 2 cups plus 2 tbsp. divided
- Sea salt to taste
- Freshly ground black pepper to taste
- Garlic – 8 cloves, roughly chopped
- Shishito peppers – 12
- Whole almonds – ½ cup, toasted and roughly chopped

- Roughly chopped parsley – 1 cup plus 1 tbsp.
- Finely grated dark chocolate – 1 tbsp.
- Sherry vinegar – 2 tsp.

Method

- Heat oven broiler. On a baking sheet, arrange cauliflower in a single layer. With 2 tbsp. of olive oil, brush both sides and season with salt and pepper. Broil for 15 minutes or until charred and tender, flipping once.
- Meanwhile, in a 12-inch nonstick skillet, heat 1 cup olive oil over medium heat. Cook garlic for 4 to 6 minutes or until golden. Transfer to a bowl and let cool.
- Whip the skillet clean and over medium-high heat, heat 1 cup of olive oil. Fry peppers for 4 to 6 minutes, or until slightly crisp and blistered. Transfer peppers to a plate lined with paper towel. Season with salt.
- Stir almonds, sherry, the chocolate, 1 cup parsley, salt and pepper into the reserved garlic oil. Then spread onto a serving platter.
- Top with cauliflower, garnish with remaining parsley and fried peppers.

# Mediterranean Breakfast Tostadas

Ingredients for 4 servings (Cook time 15 minutes)

- Tostadas – 4
- Roasted red pepper hummus – ½ cup
- Red pepper – ½ cup, diced
- Green onions -1/2 cup, chopped
- Eggs – 8, beaten

- Skim milk – ½ cup
- Garlic powder – ½ tsp.
- Oregano – ½ tsp.
- Cucumber – ½ cup, seeded and chopped
- Tomatoes – ½, diced
- Feta crumbled – ¼ cup

Method

- Place a large non-stick skillet over medium heat. Add the red peppers and cook until softened, about 2 to 3 minutes. Add green onions, oregano, garlic powder, milk, and eggs to the skillet. Stir for 2 minutes or until egg whites are no longer translucent.
- Top each tostada with tomatoes, cucumber, eggs mixture, hummus, and feta.
- Serve.

# Vanilla Chia Pudding

Ingredients for 2 to 4 servings

- Unsweetened almond milk – 2 cups
- Chia seeds – ½ cup
- Vanilla extract – 2 tsp., vanilla bean powder ½ tsp. or vanilla bean seed – 1
- Pure maple syrup or coconut – 1 tbsp., organic pure cane sugar, or turbinado, optional

Method

- In a bowl, place the ingredients and mix well. Keep in the refrigerator, covered and mix until set, or every 1 to 2 hours.
- Serve.

# Blueberry Muffins

Ingredients for 8 to 9 muffins (25 minges)

- Fine almond flour – 200 grams, about 2 cups
- Baking soda – ½ tsp.
- Fine sea salt – 1/8 tsp.
- Eggs – 3
- Honey – ¼ cup
- Ghee or coconut oil – 2 tbsp. melted
- Lemon juice – 1 tbsp.
- Organic vanilla extract – 1 tsp.
- Fresh blueberries – 1 cup

Method

- Preheat the oven to 325 F and line or grease muffin tin.
- In a large bowl, combine dry ingredients and combine wet ingredients in a medium bowl.
- Stir wet ingredients into dry ingredients and fold in the blueberries.
- Fill muffin cups ¾ cup full with a large scoop.
- Bake until golden brown and a toothpick inserted in the middle comes out clean, about 20 to 25 minutes. Cool on wire rack.
- Serve.

# Veggie Quinoa Breakfast Bowl

Ingredients for 1 serving

- Quinoa – ½ cup, rinsed
- Milk – ½ cup
- Water – ½ cup
- Cheddar cheese, grated
- Egg – 1
- Salt and pepper to taste
- Broccoli, cut into florets
- Mushrooms, sliced

Method

- In a pan, heat a little bit of olive oil over medium heat. Add mushrooms and broccoli. Stir-fry for 5 minutes or until cooked. Remove from the heat and set aside.
- In a large saucepan, combine quinoa, milk, and water. Bring to a boil and reduce heat to low. Simmer until most of the liquid is evaporated, stirring regularly.
- Add cheese, vegetables, and salt and pepper to the pot of quinoa and stir to combine. Cover and set aside.
- Fry an egg.
- Transfer the quinoa to a bowl and top with the egg.

# Buckwheat, Oat And Apple Muffins

Ingredients for 16 muffins (Cook time 18 minutes)

- Almond flour – 1 cup
- Rolled oats – 1 cup
- Buckwheat flour – 2/3 cup
- Cornstarch – 2 tbsp.
- Baking powder – 1 ½ tsp.
- Baking soda – 1 tsp.
- Ground cinnamon – 1 tsp.
- Ground cardamom – 1 tsp.
- Ground ginger – ½ tsp.
- Kosher salt – ½ tsp.
- Plain Greek yogurt – 2/3 cup
- Vegetable oil – 1/3 cup
- Pure maple syrup – 1/3 cup
- Large eggs – 3
- Unsweetened apple sauce – ¼ cup + 2 tbsp. divided
- Small apples – 3, divided (once sliced)

Method

- Preheat the oven to 400F. Line a muffin tin with cupcake liners or grease and flour it.
- To a food processor, add the ginger, cardamom, cinnamon, baking soda, baking powder, cornstarch, buckwheat flour, rolled oats, almond flour and salt. Mix on high speed until all ingredients are mixed, and oats turn into a coarse flour.
- In a medium bowl, whisk together ¼ cup of applesauce, eggs, maple syrup, vegetable oil and Greek yogurt.
- Add the dry ingredients to the wet ingredients and stir until just combined. Be careful not to over mix. Grate 2 apples and fold them into the batter.

- In the muffin pan, divide the batter and fill about half way up. In the center of each muffin, drop a tsp. of apple sauce and then top with more batter to almost fill the muffin cups. Place a few slices on top of each muffin. Press down the apples slightly.
- Bake for 18 to 20 minutes. Remove muffins to a wire rack and cool for 5 minutes.
- Serve.

# Lunch Recipes

## Crunchy Detox Salad

Ingredients for 6 servings (Cook time 30 minutes)

- Cauliflower – 2 cups
- Broccoli – 2 cups
- Red Cabbage – 1 cup, roughly chopped
- Carrots – 1 cup, roughly chopped
- Fresh parsley – 1 ½ cups
- Celery stalks – 2
- Almonds – ½ cup
- Sunflower seeds – ½ cup
- Organic raisins – 1/3 cup

For the Vinaigrette

- Olive oil – 3 tbsp.
- Lemon juice – ½ cup
- Fresh ginger – 1 tbsp. peeled and grated
- Clover honey – 2 tbsp.

- Sea salt – ½ tsp.

Method

- In a food processor, process all the ingredients until finely chopped.
- Add all the salad ingredients to a large bowl and toss with the vinaigrette.

For the vinaigrette

- In a jar with a lid, place the ingredients for the vinaigrette. Cover with a lid and shake the jar.
- Keep in the refrigerator for up to an hour and use.

# Pumpkin Lentil Soup

Ingredients for 4 servings (Cook time 30 minutes)

- Olive oil – 1 and ½ tbsp.
- Large onion – 1, peeled and chopped
- Large Potatoes – 2, peeled and chopped
- Red lentils – 4 and ½ tbsp.
- Black pepper – 1 tsp.
- Dried mint – 1 tsp.
- Cumin – ½ tsp.
- Salt – 1 ½ tsp.
- Pumpkin puree – ½ cup
- Water – 5 cups
- Lemon juice – 2 tbsp.
- Pomegranate – 2 tbsp. for garnish

- Chopped green onion – 1 tbsp. for garnish

Method

- Over medium-high heat, place a large pot. Add olive oil and chopped onions in it. Sauté until soft, about 3 to 5 minutes.
- Add in lentils and potatoes. Season with dried mint, cumin, ground black pepper, and salt. Sauté for 1 more minute and continue to stir.
- Add in the pumpkin puree and sauté for 3 more minutes.
- Pour water into the pot and let it simmer uncovered until everything is tender for about 20 minutes.
- Remove the pot from the heat and, with a hand blender, puree the soup until smooth.
- Add the lemon juice and simmer for 5 minutes more.
- Pour into serving bowls. Wait a few minutes and then garnish with chopped green onion and pomegranates.

# Black Bean Lettuce Wraps With Cilantro Lime Rice And Grilled Corn Salsa

Ingredients

- Jasmin rice – ¾ cup
- Water – 1 cup
- Black beans – 1 cup (15 ounces), rinsed and drained
- Tomato salsa – 3 tbsp.
- Juice of 1/3 lime
- Fresh Cilantro – ½ cup, chopped
- Iceberg or Bibb lettuce leaves
- Corn salsa – 1 cup

- Guacamole – ½ cup

Method

- According to package directions, prepare the jasmine rice.
- In a small pot over low heat add the beans and add tomato salsa. Stir and mix. Cook for 8 to 10 minutes, stirring occasionally.
- Add chopped cilantro to the cooked rice, then drizzle with the lime juice. Stir to combine.
- Arrange the wrap: on a serving plate, place an iceberg leaves, top with a scoop of rice, then a scoop of cooked beans and corn salsa. Sprinkle with guacamole, sliced avocado, and reserved cilantro leaves.
- Fold and enjoy.

## Quinoa-Cranberry Grilled Chicken Salad

Ingredients for 5 to 6 servings

- Chicken breasts – 3 large (about 4 lbs.)
- Garlic – 4 cloves, chopped
- Quinoa – ¾ cup
- Chopped scallions – ½ cup
- Dried cranberries – ¾ cup
- Silver almonds – ¾ cup
- Olive oil – 2 tbsp.
- Red wine vinegar – 3 tbsp.
- Balsamic vinegar – 3 tbsp.
- Honey – 1 tbsp.
- Lemon juice – ¼ cup and 1 tbsp.

- Dried sage – 1 tsp.
- Salt and pepper to taste

Method

- Cut the breasts into 3 strips each. Rub the chicken with sage, chopped garlic, and season with salt and pepper to taste. Place in a bowl with the red wine vinegar and ¼ cup of lemon juice. Cover and refrigerate for overnight.
- In a saucepan, place the quinoa and 1 ½ cups of water. Over high heat, bring to a boil and reduce to a simmer and cover. Cook until the quinoa is al dente, about 15 minutes. Place in a bowl and cool completely.
- When the chicken is ready, gill each for 6 minutes or until completely cooked through. Turn a few times for even cooking. Once cooked, immediately wrap in aluminum foil.
- When the chicken cools a bit, whisk in 1 tbsp. Lemon juice, honey, balsamic vinegar, olive oil and same salt and pepper in a bowl. Add the chopped scallions and coat them to add flavor.
- Chop the cooled chicken into 1-inch cubes. Toss the chicken with scallions, almonds, cranberries, quinoa and dressing. Add salt and pepper to taste.
- Serve.

## Tomato And White Bean Salad With Homemade Pesto And Oven-Roasted Yellow Squash

Ingredients for 1 servings (Cook time 1 hour+)

Tomato and White Bean Salad

- Organic tomatoes – 3 large, cut in eights
- White beans – 6 cups, cooked
- Extra-virgin olive oil – 2 tbsp.
- Microgreens – 4 ounces
- Pepper and sea salt to taste

Oven-roasted Yellow Squash

- Yellow squash – 3, cut into half moons
- Extra-virgin olive oil – 1 tablespoon
- Sea salt, pepper, oregano and garlic powder to taste

Basil Pesto

- Basil – 1 ½ cups
- Garlic cloves – 2
- Pine nuts – 2 tbsp.
- Juice of ½ lemon
- Extra virgin olive oil – 1/3 cup

Method

Tomato and white bean salad

- In a bowl, place the heirloom tomatoes and season with salt, toss. At 300F, oven roasts them for 30 minutes or until juicy. Let stand for 1 hour. Combine the remaining ingredients and top with micro greens. Toss gently.

Oven-roasted Yellow Squash and Pesto

- Brush the squash with olive oil and season with salt and pepper. Add garlic powder and oregano. At 375F, oven-roast for 10 to 12 minutes or until tender.

- For the pesto, in a food processor, add pine nuts, garlic cloves, basil, lemon juice and olive oil. Process for 2 minutes and add to the squash.

# Crockpot Black Bean, Sweet Potato, And Quinoa Chili

Ingredients for 8 servings

- Diced sweet potato – 3 cups (about 1 large)
- Diced red onion – 1 cup ( about 1 medium)
- Diced bell peppers – 1 cup (about 2 large)
- Garlic cloves – 3, minced
- Organic black beans – 1 (15 oz.) can
- Fire roasted tomatoes – 1 (28 oz.) can
- Vegetable broth – 3 to 4 cups
- Tomato paste – 2 tbsp.
- Uncooked quinoa – ½ cup
- Chili powder – 1 to 1 ½ tbsp.
- Cumin – 2 tsp.
- Paprika – 2 tsp.
- Coriander – 1 tsp.
- Cayenne – ½ tsp.
- Salt and pepper to taste

Method

- Add 3 cups of broth to the crockpot and add the rest of the ingredients. Turn on high and cook for 4 hours. Then, lower heat and continue to cook until ready to serve. Add ½ cup of water if the mixture is too thick.

- Serve with tortilla chips and diced avocado.

# Slow Roasted Herb Roast Beef

Ingredients for 8 servings (Cook time 1 hour)

- Eye round roast – 1.5 pound
- Garlic – 2 cloves, slivered
- Sea salt – 2 tbsp.
- Ground pepper – 1 tsp.
- Sage – 1 tsp. dried or fresh
- Oregano – 1 tsp. dried or fresh

Method

- In the fat of the roast, cut slits and insert garlic slices.
- Season roast with oregano, sage, salt and pepper. Preferably, season a day before to get more flavor.
- On the bottom of a roasting pan, place the roast with the fat and add a little water.
- Preheat the oven to 350F.
- Place in the oven until internal temperature reaches 130 to 140F on an instant-read thermometer, about 40 to 60 minutes.
- Rest the meat for 15 to 20 minutes and then carve.

# Pan-Roasted Chicken Thighs With Charred Lemon, Sage, And Rosemary

Ingredients for 8 servings (Cook time 0.46 to 1 hour)

- Pastured-raised chicken thighs – 2 pounds
- Sea salt and pepper to taste
- Organic lemons – 4 to 6, washed and quartered
- Extra virgin olive oil – 1 tbsp.
- Sage – ¼ cup
- Rosemary – ¼ cup

Method

- Heat oven to 375F.
- Season the chicken thighs with salt and pepper. Add 1 tbsp. of olive oil in a pan, add the chicken thighs, quartered lemons and season the top with rosemary and sage.
- Roast thighs until the skin is crisp to your liking and chicken is cooked through, about 35 to 45 minutes.
- Before serving, squeeze a wedge of lemon on the chicken and serve.

## Beef Stir Fry With Onions And Peppers

Ingredients for 8 servings (5 to 10 minutes)

- Grass fed flank steak – 1 pound, cut into strips
- Balsamic vinegar – 2 tsp.
- Rice wine – 1 tbsp.
- Extra virgin olive oil – 3 tbsp.
- Large yellow onion – 1, sliced into thin strips
- Green bell pepper – ½, sliced into thin strips

- Red bell pepper – ½, sliced into thin strips
- Sea salt and pepper to taste
- Crushed red pepper flakes
- Sesame seeds

Method

- Place the strips in a bowl. Add rice wine and vinegar, salt and pepper, toss.
- On high heat, heat pan and add 1 tbsp of olive oil. Add the beef and cook until the beef brown a bit, about 20 to 30 seconds. Then stir the beef for 2 minutes more.
- Remove beef and place aside. Now, add the remaining 1 tsp. of oil to the pan and add the onions. Stir and cook for 2 minutes or until caramelized. Add the peppers and cook for 2 minutes more. Return beef to pan and add sesame seeds and red pepper flakes. If the sauce is too thin, add 1 tsp. of corn starch.

# Pork Adobado

Ingredients for 9 servings (Cook time 1+ hour)

- Dried New Mexico chilies – 5 ounces, steamed
- Ancho chili – 1 tbsp. Fresh or powder
- Pasilla chilies – 1 tbsp.
- Guajillo chilies – ½ tbsp.
- Mexican chili powder – ½ tbsp.
- White wine vinegar – 1 tbsp.
- Ground cumin – 2 tsp.
- Cayenne pepper – 1/8 tsp.

- Juice of 1 orange
- Extra-virgin olive oil – 5 tbsp.
- Boneless pork shoulder or pork stew meat – 3 pounds, cut into 1 ½ inch chunks
- Yellow onion – 1, diced
- Sea salt and ground pepper to taste

Method

- In a large pot, heat all the chilies over medium-high heat for 5 minutes. Transfer them to a large bowl and add 8 cups of boiling water. Set aside for 15 to 20 minutes.
- Drain chiles and reserve 1 to 2 cups of the liquid. Add the remaining spices including cayenne, cumin, chili powder, pepper, salt, juice of an orange, vinegar, and reserve liquid.
- Puree until smooth.
- Place the pan over medium-high heat and add oil to the pot.
- Season pork with salt and pepper and brown the pork on all sides.
- Add the sauce to the pan. Reduce the heat to low, cover and cook for 1 ½ hours or until pork is tender, stirring occasionally. Add some diced onions at the 45-minute mark.

# Dinner Recipes

## Butternut Squash And Wild Rice Salad With Balsamic Dressing

Ingredients for 6 servings

Dressing

- Extra-virgin olive oil or sunflower oil – ¼ cup
- Pure maple syrup – 2 tbsp.
- Balsamic vinegar – 2 tbsp.
- Sea salt – ½ tsp.
- Black pepper – scant ½ tsp.
- Chopped fresh rosemary – ½ tbsp.
- Garlic – 1 clove, minced

Salad

- Peeled and finely chopped butternut squash – 2 ½ cups
- Olive oil – 1 ½ tbsp.
- Sea salt and black pepper to taste
- Thinly sliced kale or spinach – 2 ½ cups
- Thinly sliced leeks – ½ cup, both green and white parts
- Dried cranberries or cherries – ½ cup
- Thinly sliced fresh basil – ¼ cup
- Cooked wild rice – 3 cups, warmed

Method

- Preheat the oven to 400F. In a bowl, add squash and drizzle with olive oil, season with salt and pepper, toss.
- Spread onto a baking sheet and roast until fork tender, about 25 minutes, stirring once.
- In a large bowl, combine basil, cherries, leeks and spinach.
- Stir in squash and warm rice, so the squash wilts mildly from the heat.
- Stir dressing into the salad. Taste and adjust seasoning.
- Serve.

To make the sauce

- Puree all ingredients with an immersion blender.

# Sweet Potato Kale Lentil Soup

Ingredients for 6 to 7 servings

- Green lentils – 2 cups
- Vegetable stock – 5 to 7 cups
- Small carrots – 3, chopped
- Sweet Potatoes – 2 small, cubed
- Onion – 1, chopped
- Garlic – 2 to 3 cloves, minced
- Bay leaf – 1
- Dried thyme – ½ tsp.
- Sea salt to taste
- Kale – 3 leaves, stems separated and roughly chopped

Method

- Except for the kale, place all the ingredients in a large stock pot.
- Bring to a boil, then cover. Lower heat and simmer for 30 minutes or until lentils are soft.
- Add kale during the last 5 minutes of cooking.
- Serve.

# Quinoa Salad And Lime Orange Dressing

Ingredients for 2 to 3 servings (Cook time 15 minutes)

Salad

- Mixed Greens – 5 to 6 cups
- Cooked Quinoa – 1 cup
- Fresh or canned corn – ½ cup
- Cooked black beans – 1 cup (seasoned with garlic powder, chili, cumin, and sea salt)
- Red onion – ¼ cup, diced
- Orange – 1, segmented
- Ripe avocado – ½, chopped
- Fresh Cilantro – ¼ cup, chopped or torn

Dressing

- Ripe avocado – ½
- Large lime – 1, juiced
- Orange juice – 3 tbsp.
- Hot sauce – 1 to 2 tsp.
- Cumin powder – ¼ tsp.
- Chili powder – 1/8 tsp.
- Pinch of sea salt and black powder
- Fresh minced cilantro – 1 tbsp.
- Extra virgin olive oil or avocado oil – 3 to 4 tbsp.

Method

- Prepare salad ingredients by warming black beans, segmenting the orange, chopping vegetables and seasoning with garlic powder, chili, cumin, and salt.

- Add all dressing ingredients to a food process and blend until smooth and creamy. Scrape down sides as needed. Adjust seasoning if needed.
- Place salad and serve with dressing on the side.

# Vegan Chickpea, Cauliflower, And Potato Curry

Ingredients

- Cauliflower – 1 large (2 lbs.) head, trimmed
- Yukon gold potatoes – ¾ lb.
- Vegetable oil – 2 tbsp.
- Medium onions – 3, chopped
- Garlic – 4 cloves, minced
- Fresh ginger – 1-pinch, peeled and finely grated
- Ground coriander – 2 tsp.
- Ground cumin – 2 tsp.
- Ground cardamom – ¼ tsp.
- Dried red pepper flakes – 1 pinch
- Star anise – 2
- Chopped tomatoes – 1 ( 28-ounce) can
- Chickpeas – 1 (14 to 15 ounce) can, drained and rinsed
- Vegetable broth – 2 cups
- Garam masala – 1 tbsp.
- Light coconut milk – ¾ cup
- Large bunch of fresh cilantro, chopped
- Kosher salt and freshly ground pepper

Method

- Chop the potatoes into ¾-inch chunks and cut the cauliflower into medium-sized florets. Place the potatoes and cauliflower in a large pot and fill with cold water. Add a generous amount of salt and bring to a rolling boil over medium-high heat. Remove from heat and drain into a colander. Set aside and keep the potatoes and cauliflowers warm.
- In a large heavy pot, heat the oil and add the ginger, garlic, and onions. Sauté until the onions are very soft and translucent, about 8 to 10 minutes, stirring every few minutes. Adjust heat if necessary.
- Add star anise, salt, pepper, red pepper flakes, cardamom, cumin, coriander and cook until very fragrant, about 2 to 3 minutes, stirring frequently. Add drained chickpeas and tomatoes with their juices. Stir and mix. Add the potatoes, cauliflower and the vegetable broth. Bring the mixture to a low simmer and simmer until potatoes and cauliflowers are fork tender, about 10 minutes, stirring occasionally.
- Stir in coconut milk and garam masala, simmer for 10 minutes more. Season to taste with salt and pepper.
- Sprinkle with roughly chopped cilantro and serve with naan or rice.

## Lemon Chicken Stew

Ingredients for 6 to 8 servings

- Canola oil – 5 tbsp.
- All-purpose flour – ½ cup
- Kosher salt and freshly ground pepper
- Skinless and boneless chicken thighs – 1 pound, cut into 1-inch pieces
- Carrots – 4, sliced

- Celery – 2 ribs, chopped
- Onion – 1, diced
- Leek – 1, thinly sliced
- Garlic – 2 cloves, minced
- Chicken stock – 5 cups
- Water – 1 cup
- Lemon juice – 3 tbsp.
- Orzo pasta – 1 cup
- Fresh tarragon – 2 tbsp. chopped

Method

- Heat 2 tbsp. of oil in an 8-quart casserole stockpot over medium-high heat. To a shallow bowl, add the flour and season with about 1 tsp. each of pepper and kosher salt.
- Coat the chicken in flour and shake off the excess. Place ½ of the chicken in the stockpot but don't overfill. Cook 2 minutes per side, or until golden brown and transfer to a bowl. Repeat with the rest of the chicken.
- Add the remaining 1 tbsp. of oil and onion, celery and carrots to the stock pot and cook for 3 minutes on medium heat. Add the garlic and sliced leek and cook for 2 minutes and season with salt and pepper. Add the water and chicken stock and bring to a boil.
- Cover and simmer over low heat for 20 minutes. Stirring occasionally. Add the chicken and orzo to the stockpot and simmer until orzo is tender about 10 minutes. Stir in lemon juice, sprinkle with tarragon, and season with salt and pepper.

# Quinoa, Sweet Potato, And Black Bean Burger

Ingredients for 4 servings

For the veggie burgers

- Sweet Potatoes – 3 to 4 (3/4 lb.), cut in half lengthwise
- Chopped white onion – ¾ cup
- Minced garlic – 1 tbsp.
- Jalapeno pepper – 1, seeds removed and diced
- Black beans – 1 (15.5) can, rinsed and drained
- All-purpose flour – ¼ cup
- Smoked paprika – 1 tsp.
- Garlic powder – 1 tsp.
- Cooked Quinoa – 1 cup
- Olive oil salt

For the avocado spread

- Avocado – 1, pit removed
- Cilantro leaves – 1/8 cup
- Garlic – 1 clove, chopped
- Salt – ½ tsp.
- White wine vinegar – 2 tsp.

For the slaw

- Thinly sliced red cabbage – 1 cup
- Rice wine vinegar – 2 tbsp.
- Salt – to taste
- Hamburger buns – 4

For the veggie burgers

- Preheat the oven to 375F and line a baking sheet with aluminum foil.

- On the baking sheet, place sweet potato halves and drizzle with 1 ½ tbsp olive oil and sprinkle with kosher salt. Cook for 30 minutes. Flip once halfway through.
- Meanwhile, in a skillet heat 2 tsp. olive oil over medium heat. Add garlic and onion and season with ½ tsp. salt. Cook for 2 minutes, then lower heat and cook for 3 minutes more. Stirring occasionally. Remove from the heat and set aside.
- Once the sweet potato is cooked, remove from the oven. Cool and then peel the skin. Place in a bowl and mash with a fork.
- Stir in chopped jalapeno, onion and garlic.
- Mix in black beans, then add smoked paprika, garlic powder, and flour. Once they are mixed, mix in the quinoa.
- Line a plate with parchment paper. Take ¼ cup of mixture and make patties. Place on a lined plate and repeat with the remaining mixture. Refrigerate patties for 30 minutes.
- In a medium skillet, heat 1 tbsp. of olive oil over medium-high heat. Add burgers and cook until brown, about 3 to 4 minutes on each side.
- Line a baking sheet with aluminum foil and place the cooked patties on it. In the 375F oven, cook the patties for 15 to 20 minutes. Flip half way through.

For the avocado spread

- With an immersion blender, puree the garlic, cilantro, avocado, white wine vinegar and ½ tsp salt until smooth.

For the slaw

- Toss the sliced red cabbage with salt, rice wine vinegar and let sit for 10 minutes.

Arranging the burger

- On top of the bottom half of the bun, place two veggie burgers. Top with slow. On the top half of the bun, spread avocado mixture, and place on top of the slaw.
- Serve.

# California Avocado, Veggie, Rice And Chicken Bowls

Ingredients (Cook time 25 minutes)

Chicken

- Boneless skinless chicken breast or tenders – 1 pound ( cubed if using skewers)
- Olive oil – ¼ cup
- Garlic – 4 cloves, minced
- Onion powder – ½ tsp.
- Pepper – ½ tsp.
- Cayenne – ¼ tsp.
- Smoked paprika – ½ tsp.
- Fresh parsley – ¼ cup, chopped
- Fresh basil – ¼ cup, chopped

The rice + veggies + avocado

- Jasmin or basmati rice – 1 ½ cups, cooked
- Water – 3 cups
- Red pepper – 2, cut into fourths
- Zucchini – 1 inch, sliced into ¼ rounds
- Olive oil – 1 tbsp.

- Salt and pepper
- Avocados – 2, mashed very well
- Juice of 1 lemon
- Fresh parsley – ½ cup , chopped
- Garlic – 1 clove, minced
- Salt and pepper to taste
- Grape Tomatoes – 1 pint, halved
- Walnuts – ¼ cup, toasted
- Blue cheese – ½ cup, crumbled

Method

- If you're using bamboo skewers, soak them in water for 30 minutes before grilling.
- In a large bowl, combine the basil, parsley, smoked paprika, cayenne, pepper, onion powder, garlic, and olive oil. Add the chicken and toss well. Keep in the refrigerator and prepare the rest.
- Preheat the grill to medium-high heat.
- To a gallon size zip lock bag, add the zucchini and red pepper. Season with salt and pepper and drizzle with 1 tbsp olive oil. Seal the bag and shake well so the oil coats the veggies.
- Remove the chicken from the fridge and skewer the chicken.
- Grill the chicken 3 to 4 minutes per side. Rotate several times until chicken has light char marks and chicken is cooked through.
- Meanwhile, grill the zucchini until tender, about 4 minutes on each side. Grill the red peppers for 5 minutes, and rotate a few times while grilling. Or you can cook everything on the stove.

- Remove everything from the grill and let cool for 5 minutes. Slice the cooled red peppers into strips.
- To a bowl, add the mashed avocados. Stir in garlic, parsley, lemon juice and season with salt and pepper to taste. Mix well.
- Divide the rice among 4 plates. Top each plate of rice with equal amounts of zucchini, peppers, and chicken. Add mashed avocado and then add the walnuts and fresh tomatoes.
- Sprinkle with blue cheese and serve.

# Kale Soup

Ingredients for 4 servings (Cook time 16 to 30 minutes)

- Extra-virgin olive oil – 2 tbsp.
- Garlic – 2 to 4 cloves, diced
- Small Potatoes – 4, peeled and diced
- Butternut squash – ½, diced
- Large yellow onion – 1, chopped
- Spicy chorizo – ½ pound
- Chicken bone broth – 1 quart
- Fresh kale – ¾ pounds, washed, stems removed and shredded
- Tomato – 1, diced
- Bay leaf – 1
- Sea salt and freshly ground pepper to taste

Method

- In a deep pot, heat olive oil over medium heat. Add onions, butternut squash, and potatoes. Cover and cook for 5 minutes. Stir if necessary.
- Add kale, bay leaf, and garlic. Cover for 2 minutes, or until the greens are wilted. Add salt and pepper.
- Add the broth, chorizo, and tomatoes. Bring the mixture to a full boil for 2 minutes. Then lower the heat and simmer for about 15 to 20 minutes until potatoes are tender .

# Spaghetti Squash, Sausage And Kale Boats

Ingredients for 4 servings

- Spaghetti squash – 1 medium or 2 small
- Italian chicken sausage – 1 ½ lbs. casings removed
- Yellow onion – 1, diced
- Garlic – 4 cloves, minced
- Kale – 1 bunch
- Extra virgin olive oil – 3 tbsp. plus more for drizzling
- Salt and pepper
- Pine nuts – 2 tbsp. roasted
- Fresh parsley – 2 tbsp. chopped

Method

- Preheat the oven to 400F.
- In the microwave, place the squash for 3 to 4 minutes to soften.
- Cut the squash with a sharp knife in half lengthwise. Scoop out the seeds and discard. On a rimmed baking sheet, place

the halves with the cut side up. Sprinkle with salt, pepper and drizzle with olive oil.

- Roast in the oven until you can poke the squash with a fork, about 45 to 50 minutes. Set aside to cool.
- Meanwhile, prepare the kale by cutting up the leaves and removing the center stems. In a large skillet, heat the olive oil over medium heat. Add the garlic and onion and sauté for 4 to 5 minutes. Add the sausage and use a spatula to break it apart.
- Cook until the sausage is cooked through and browned, about 10 to 12 minutes. Stirring regularly. Add the kale and stir. Cook until the kale wilts. Remove from heat and set aside.
- Use a fork to scrape the insides of the spaghetti squash and shred the squash into strands. Add the strands into the skillet with the sausage and toss to combine. Season with salt and pepper.
- Divide the mixture into squash shells, top with parsley and pine nuts and serve.

# Greek Turkey Burgers

Ingredients for 6 servings

- Plain Greek yogurt – 7 oz.
- Fresh lemon – 1 medium
- Minced Garlic – ¼ tsp.
- Dried dill – ¼ tsp.
- Ground Turkey – 1.25 lb.
- Sun dried tomatoes – 6, halves
- Red onion – 1 medium
- Frozen spinach – 2 oz.

70

- Crumbled feta – ¼ cup
- Dried oregano – 1 tsp.
- Minced Garlic – ½ tsp.
- Breadcrumbs – 1/3 cup
- Egg – 1 large
- Cucumber – 1 medium
- Hamburger buns – 6
- Salt and pepper to taste

Method


- Prepare the yogurt sauce by combining the juice of half the lemon, salt, dry dill, ¼ tsp minced garlic, and yogurt. Mix everything and keep in the refrigerator until time to use.
- Thaw the frozen spinach and squeeze moisture as much as possible. Roughly chop the spinach.
- In a bowl, combine the egg, bread crumbs, ground pepper, ½ tsp salt, dried oregano, ½ tsp minced garlic, feta, red onion, sun-dried tomatoes, ground turkey, and spinach. Mix everything and shape the mixture into 6 patties.
- In a non-stick skillet, cook the burgers.
- To assemble: on both sides of a bun, spread the yogurt sauce add a warm burger and top with cucumber and red onion. Serve.

# Snacks

## Dill Crackers


Ingredients for 3 to 4 dozen crackers

- Eggs – 3
- Ghee or coconut oil – 3 tbsp.
- Cold water – 6 tbsp.
- Onion powder – 1 tsp.
- Granulated garlic – 1 tsp.
- Chopped fresh dill – 1 tsp.
- Sea salt – ½ tsp.
- Black pepper – ½ tsp.
- Arrowroot flour – 2 tbsp.
- Coconut flour – 1 cup

Method

- In a bowl, whisk together the dill, salt, pepper, granulated garlic, onion powder, water, ghee, and eggs. Sift the coconut flour and arrowroot flour into the wet mixture and combine until incorporated. Make 2 balls with the mixture and wrap each ball tightly with plastic wrap. Keep in the refrigerator for 20 minutes to chill.
- Preheat the oven to 350F.
- With a rolling pin, roll the chilled balls between 2 sheets of parchment paper one by one until they are an even 1/8 inch thick rectangle.
- Transfer the sheet to 2 separate sheet pans and slice into crackers.
- Bake until the edges of the crackers are golden brown, about 10 to 12 minutes.

# Buttermilk Buns

Ingredients for 8 buns

- Full-fat coconut milk – ¼ cup, canned
- Apple cider vinegar – 1 tbsp.
- Gelatin – 2 tsp.
- Egg – 4, cold
- Coconut flour – ¼ cup, sifted
- Almond flour – ¼ cup
- Baking soda – 1 tsp.
- Sea salt – ½ tsp.

Method

- Preheat the oven to 350F and line a baking sheet with parchment paper.
- In a bowl, whisk gelatin, apple cider vinegar, and coconut milk and let it sit for 5 minutes.
- In another bowl, whisk together the salt, baking soda, almond flour, coconut flour, coconut milk mixture, and eggs. Let sit for 5 minutes.
- Onto the prepared baking sheet, scoop 3 tbsp of the batter and gently spread it into 3-inch circles.
- Bake until the buns feel springy in the center when gently pressed, about 10 to 15 minutes.

# Celery Root Cakes

Ingredients for 12 small cakes

- Egg – 1
- Sea salt – ½ tsp.
- Black pepper – ½ tsp.

- Granulated garlic – ½ tsp.
- Celery root – 1 large, peeled and shredded (2 cups)
- Coconut oil for pan frying

Method

- Whisk the egg with seasonings in a large bowl. Add the celery root and mix together until celery root is well coated.
- In a large skillet, melt enough coconut oil or cooking fat to cover the enter bottom of your skillet in a very thin layer.
- Take 2 tbsp. of the mixture and make a loose ball and press into a thin, even layer in the bottom of the skillet. Repeat with the rest of the mixture.
- Fry for 1 minute or until browned on one side, then flip and cook 1 minute more on the other side. Repeat with the rest of the mixture. Transfer on a paper lined plate.

## Sundried Tomato Hummus

Ingredients for 2 cups

- Cauliflower florets – 4 cups, steamed
- Sesame tahini – 2 tbsp. plus more if desired
- Extra-virgin olive oil – ¼ cup plus 1 tbsp.
- Small clove garlic – 1, minced
- Zest and juice of 1 lemon
- Pinch of ground cumin
- Salt and pepper to taste
- Sundried tomatoes – 6, plus more for garnish
- Paprika for garnish

Method

- In a food processor, combine the cumin, lemon juice, garlic, ¼-cup olive oil, tahini and cauliflower and process until smooth. Add the sundried tomatoes and pulse to combine.
- Remove from the food processor and garnish with additional diced sundried tomatoes, a sprinkling of paprika, 1 tbsp. of olive oil, and lemon zest.
- Serve with olive and sliced fresh vegetables.

## Smoky Lime Nut Mix

Ingredients for 1 ½ cup

- Raw almonds – ½ cup
- Raw walnuts – ½ cup
- Raw pecans – ½ cup
- Juice of ½ lime
- Coconut oil 1 ½ tbsp. melted
- Smoky spice blend – 2 tbsp.
- Sea salt to taste
- Zest of 1 lime

Method

- Preheat the oven to 275F.
- In a bowl, combine the lime juice and nuts and toss to coat. Let sit for 5 minutes.
- In another bowl, combine the lime zest, spice blend and melted coconut oil.

- Toss the nuts in the lime juice one more time to cat. Then, drain the excess lime juice from the bowl.
- Add the coconut oil mixture and toss to coat the mixed nuts. Season with salt to taste.
- On a rimmed baking sheet, spread the nuts out in a single layer and bake until toasted, about 20 to 25 minutes.
- Place a glass jar and keep in the refrigerator.

# Kale Chips

Ingredients for 4 to 6 servings

- Coconut oil – 3 tbsp. melted
- Almond or other nut or seed meal – ½ cup
- Nutritional yeast – ½ cup
- Apple cider vinegar – ¼ cup
- Sea salt – 1 tsp.
- Kale – 1 large bunch (rinsed, dried, steam removed and large leaves cut into smaller pieces)

Method

- Preheat the oven to 350F.
- In a bowl, combine the salt, vinegar, nutritional yeast, almond meal, and coconut oil.
- Place the kale in the bowl with topping mixture. Rub the mixture into the kale leaves.
- Then, spread the kale in a single layer on a baking sheet.
- Bake until the kale becomes crispy but not browned, about 15 to 20 minutes. If the kale is still a bit soggy after 20

minutes, then turn off the oven and keep the kale in the oven for 20 minutes more.

# Turkey Jerky

Ingredients for 8 servings

- Skinless, boneless turkey breast – 2 pounds (frozen for couple of hours)
- Coconut aminos – ½ cup
- Fish sauce – 1 tbsp.
- Chines five spice powder – ½ tsp.
- Sea salt – 1 tsp.

Method

- Whisk the ingredients together for the marinade. Taste and adjust seasonings as needed.
- Remove the turkey breast from the freezer and cut into thin slices.
- Place the sliced meat in the marinade and keep in the refrigerator overnight.
- Preheat the oven to 200F.
- On top of 2 foil-lined rimmed baking sheets, place oven-safe baking racks.
- Remove the meat from the refrigerator and place the racks ½ inch apart.
- Bake until the jerky reaches the desired level of dryness, about 3 to 4 hours.

# Coconut Chia Seed Pudding

Ingredients for 1 serving

- Coconut water – 1 cup
- Chia seeds – 3 tbsp.
- Vanilla powder – 1 tsp.
- Ground cinnamon – 1 tsp.

Method

- Combine all the ingredients together and keep the mixture in the refrigerator overnight.
- Serve.

## Avocado With Poppy Seeds And Lemon

Ingredients for 1 serving

- Avocado – ½ (cut in half and pit removed)
- Juice of ¼ lemon
- Poppy seeds – ½ tsp.
- Pinch of unrefined salt

Method

- Drizzle the avocado with lemon juice, sprinkle with salt and poppy seeds.
- Serve.

## Juicy Green Booster

Ingredients for 1 serving

- Spinach – 8 ¾ oz.
- Kale - 8 ¾ oz.
- Carrot – 1, peeled
- Celery – 1 stalk
- English cucumber – 1
- Lemon – 1, peeled
- Fresh ginger – 1 1/5 inch

Method

- Cup up all the vegetables.
- Blend in a blender and serve.

# Chapter 10: Life Without Sugar

Once you quit sugar, your mental and physical health will transform within weeks. People who have successfully quit sugar tell us what actually quitting sugar means:

- It means a life without processed foods: When you eliminate sugar from your diet, you basically eliminate everything that comes in a box or a packet. The most important rule of quitting sugar is not eating any processed foods.
- It means eating like your ancestors: Quitting sugar means eating, real, whole foods that don't contain additives, preservatives, and other chemicals. Eat how your grandparents used to eat.

Here is how dieters feel after they quit sugar. They attest to the following from their experience:

- You will lose weight: After completing the sugar diet, most of the dieters lost weight. They looked more attractive, had flatter bellies, felt great and didn't have those annoying fluid retention or bloating problem.
- Improved skin: Sugar creates AGEs or harmful advanced glycation end-products and accelerates your aging process. Sugar makes elastin and collagen less elastic, radiant, supple, resilient and more prone to sun damage. Within a few weeks of quitting sugar, your skin will improve, and you will have glowing, healthy skin again.
- You will eat better: You avoid eating sugar and focus on eating real, whole and unprocessed foods. The main goal of quitting sugar is to bring back your natural appetite. You will naturally eat fewer calories and avoid overeating.
- You have more self-control: Self-control is a limited resource, so you need to manage it very carefully. When you quit

sugar, you don't have to self-control when it comes to eating. Instead, you can focus your self-control on matters like career and relationships.

- You will heal your thyroid: Often thyroid related problems cause you to gain weight and heighten your risk of developing high cholesterol and diabetes. Once you quit sugar, you solve any thyroid related problem and avoid these conditions.

Here are some other positive things life offers you when you quit sugar:

- Your food will taste better, especially fruit: Fruit is delicious and sweet with natural, healthy sugar. Once you quit sugar, you will truly enjoy the sweet taste of sugar.

- More sensitive taste buds: Eating sugar rich foods dulls your taste buds. So once you quit sugar, your taste-buds will improve. You will enjoy all the natural sweets nature has to offer and understand that you only need natural sugars and don't have to add any added sugar to your meals.

- You will enjoy eating whole foods as snacks: Foods like Pellegrino, Medjool dates, no added sugar crackers, and new brands of spaghetti sauce will replace your sugar-rich snacks, and you will enjoy them more.

- The upward spiral: Once you quit sugar, your diet choices become healthier. Day after day, you eat healthy, whole foods and the upward spiral continuous.

- Feeling better, all round: You will feel great both mentally and physically.

# Chapter 11: 10 Low Carb Ice Creams

## 1) Chocolate And Peanut Butter Ice Cream!

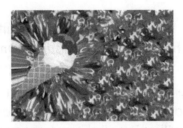

This recipe is surprisingly low in carbs; it is sugar free and even gluten free!

**Ingredients:**

- Almond milk
- Cottage Cheese
- Whipping Cream
- Egg
- Vanilla extract
- Stevia extract
- Natural Peanut Butter
- Glucomannan
- Coconut Oil
- Cocoa powder

You can mix these ingredients by hand or in a home ice cream maker.Simply place 2 cups of almond milk, with½cup cottage cheese,½cup whipping cream, the egg, a teaspoon of vanilla, a tablespoon of stevia and a teaspoon of glucomannan into your bowl.Then blend them thoroughly.

Separately you can mix¼cup coconut oil, two tablespoons of cocoa powder and a teaspoon of stevia.This can then be gently heated on the stove to melt it.

The original mixture needs to be put into a suitable container and placed into the freezer.Once it has been in there for five minutes you can bring it back out.Place two spoons of peanut butter on top of the ice cream and the liquid chocolate.Then mix it together; swirling it through the ice cream.Your finished product can then go back into the freezer until it has finished freezing!

## 2) Chocolate Ice Cream

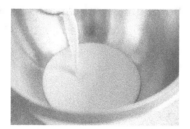

**Ingredients**

- Heavy cream
- Unsweetened Cashew milk

- Cocoa powder
- Stevia
- Egg Yolks
- Dark chocolate
- Vanilla extract

To make this ice cream you will need to put a bowl over an ice bath.You can then mix the two cups of the cream with a cup of cashew milk and two large tablespoons of cocoa powder in a pan.It is also worth adding a tablespoon of stevia.You will need to blend this mixture and heat until it reaches 170F

In a separate bowl you will need to place your four egg yolks and pour one cup of the hot mixture in with them.You will need to whisk the mixture continuously as you do so.You can then pour this mixture into the original mixture and mix it again.

The pan can then go back on the stove; keep stirring until the mixture reaches 175F.Whilst still hot add 3oz of chopped dark chocolate; preferably at least 70%.

Leave the mixture to sit for five minutes and then whisk smooth.It can then be put into your ice bath bowl and leave to cool. It can then be wrapped in cling film and placed into the freezer.It must be left in there for at least three hours

After three hours add½cup cashew milk and½teaspoon of vanilla extract; whisk it thoroughly; you can use an ice cream maker if you like!It can be eaten straight away or placed back into the freezer until required.

# 3) Sugar Free Peanut Butter Ice Cream

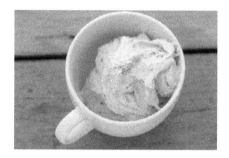

**Ingredients**

- Unsweetened almond milk

- Natural peanut butter

- Cream cheese

- Stevia

- Vanilla extract

Photo made by: Jules

Creating this ice cream is simple!Simply add 2½cups of almond milk to½cup peanut butter, 8 oz cream cheese and one teaspoon of vanilla extract.You will also need a tablespoon of stevia.

Then blend all the ingredients for several minutes to ensure they are well mixed.You can taste it at this stage and adjust any part of the recipe you need to.

Once blended, add to an ice cream maker and churn for approximately twenty minutes.Then place into a freezer container and freeze!It should be ready to eat in approximately one hour.

# 4) Avocado Sorbet

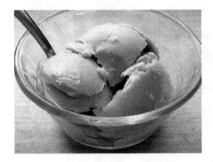

Photo made by: Joy

**Ingredients**

- Almond milk

- Avocados

- Stevia

- Lime juice

- Sea salt

Simply mix 2 cups of almond milk with two avocados, a large tablespoon of stevia and a tablespoon of lime juice.You can also add¼teaspoon of sea salt to help keep the sorbet soft.All these items should be blended in a food processor until smooth.Then simply add to your ice cream maker and churn for fifteen minutes.It can then be transferred to a freezer container and frozen!You can defrost and refreeze this as many times as you like!

# 5) Peanut Butter Sticks

**Ingredients**

- Heavy Cream

- Almond Milk–unsweetened
- Vanilla extract
- Natural peanut butter
- Stevia

Start by whipping one cup of heavy cream until you can create soft peaks which stay.You can then continue to whisk whilst adding one¾cup of almond milk,¾cup of peanut butter; two teaspoons of vanilla and ¼cup stervia.

You will need to whisk for approximately five minutes to get stiff peaks.You can then pour the mixture into molds; these can be any shape you like!You will need to add sticks to hold them with before you place them into the freezer.

The ice creams should be ready in approximately three hours to enjoy!

# 6) Coconut Ice Cream

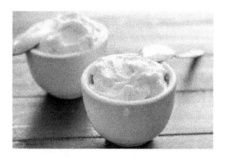

Photo made by: Jules

**Ingredients**

- Eggs
- Vanilla extract

- Lime Juice

- Butter

- Coconut Oil

- XCT Oil

- Erythritol

- Water

You will need a blender to create this delicious ice cream.Simply mix four eggs with two teaspoons of vanilla extract, five drops of lime juice and one cup of butter.You also need to add a cup of coconut oil, half a cup of XCT oil and¾cup of Erythritol.

Blend all of these until your mixture is creamy.You can then add up to a cup of water; but add a little at a time until you get a smooth consistency.You will then be ready to put it into your ice cream maker follow the instructions which come with your machine!

## 7) Lemon Poppy Seed Ice Cream

### Ingredients

- Coconut Milk

- Chia Seeds

- Stevia

- Poppy Seeds

- Lemon Juice

- Coconut oil

You can choose whether to add the poppy seeds at the start of the recipe to ensure a smooth ice cream, or at the end to add a little crunch.

You will need to grind a¼cup of chia seeds and, if desired, two tablespoons of poppy seeds.You can then blend the ground seeds with 3 cups of coconut milk.You will then need to add¼cup lemon juice,½teaspoon stevia and¼cup coconut oil.

Give the mixture a quick stir and then freeze it.As soon as it is frozen you can remove it and cut it into chunks.You will then be able to blend it and refreeze it.This avoids the need to have an ice cream maker!

# 8) Mint Fudge Ice Cream

Despite being an unusual mix of flavors this is one delicious treat!

**Ingredients**

- Almond Milk
- Spinach
- Stevia
- Cottage Cheese
- Whipping Cream
- Mint extract
- Sea Salt
- Glucomannan

The fudge requires making; to ensure it is sugar free and low carb.Its ingredients are:

- Dark chocolate
- Coconut oil
- Butter
- Stevia
- Almond milk

You can make the ice cream with virtually no effort.Simply mix 1 cup almond milk with½cup fresh spinach,¼cup cottage cheese and¼cup whipping cream.

You will also need to add¼teaspoon of stevia, 1 teaspoon of glucomannan and¼teaspoon of mint extract.The mixed ingredients should be placed in a blender until the mixture is smooth.Then simply add it to your ice cream maker and follow its instructions.

Whilst the ice cream maker is working you can mix½ oz dark chocolate with½tablespoon of butter and½a tablespoon of coconut oil.Then add a pinch of stevia and a tablespoon of almond milk. Microwave this mixture on a low power stopping regularly to stir, until it is all melted.

Once the ice cream has frozen you can drizzle this fudge mix across the top.Either eat it immediately or stick it back into the freezer until you want it!

# 9) Frozen Yoghurt Ice Cream

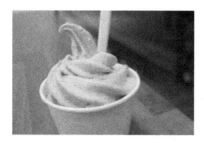

Strictly speaking it may be difficult to call this an ice cream.However, it can be enjoyed as one and is too delicious to leave out of the book!

Photo made by: stu_spivack

**Ingredients:**

- Frozen berries of your choice

- Plain Yoghurt

- Almond milk

- Ice

- Stevia–can be almond flavor if you prefer!

To create this delicious treat you can simply blend two cups of berries with one cup of plain yoghurt and½cup of almond milk.You will also need to add a cup of ice and a teaspoon of stevia.

Once the mixture is fully blended simply put it into your ice cream maker and follow the instructions on your machine.Alternatively you can freeze it in a suitable container for several hours.For those who are not concerned with sugar or carb content it is possible to add any sauce you wish to your ice cream dessert.

# 10) Coffee Ice Cream

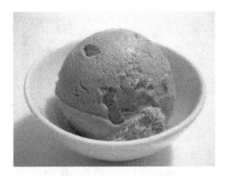

**Photo made by: gordonramsaysubmissions**

This is another ice cream which can be made without the aid of an ice cream maker.

**Ingredients**

- Heavy cream
- Almond milk
- Stevia
- Butter
- Xanthan Gum
- Instant coffee
- Vanilla extract

The first step is to place one cup of cream into a saucepan with one cup of almond milk.This mixture needs to be brought to boiling point and then allowed to simmer for approximately one hour.

You can then remove the pan from the stove and add a tablespoon of stevia and one tablespoon of butter.Whisk this until smooth before adding¼teaspoon of xanthan gum and 2 tablespoons of your favorite instant coffee; along with¼teaspoon of vanilla extract.Whisk it until the coffee has dissolved and then leave the mixture to cool.

In a separate bowl, whisk 1½cups of heavy whipping cream until it holds its peaks. You can then fold in your pan of mixture before pouring the entire mix into a suitable container and freezing.It should be ready in approximately six hours.

# Chapter 12: 10 Low Carb Slushies

## 1) The Fruit Slushy

This fresh and light slushy will leave you feeling great!

**Ingredients:**

- Chopped Fresh fruit of your choice

- Ice

- Sparkling water

Start by washing chopping and, if necessary, de-seeding your fruit.You need 1½cups of chopped fruit.Place the fruit into your blender and add one cup of ice and¼cup sparkling water.Now blend it until it reaches your desired consistency and then pour into a glass before you enjoy!

If you wish you can add a little lemon juice or similar to adjust the flavor; this should be done before it is blended.

## 2) The Coke Slushy

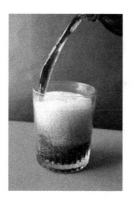

Fortunately this version of the coke slushy is actually sugar free!

**Ingredients**

- Sugar free Coca Cola

- Ice

- Lime

Simply mix one liter of sugar free Coke with 2½cups of ice in your blender.Next you will need to pulse the blender until your mixture has reached the required consistency; then pour it into two glasses.Take one lime and cut it into quarters.One quarter can be squeezed into each drink; the remaining two quarters can be placed on each glass to create the right look.

Then sit back and enjoy!

## 3) Kool-Aid Slushy

This type of slushy is usually laden with sugar; but it is possible to do it without!

**Ingredients**

- Sugar Free soda

- Unsweetened Kool-Aid mix

- Ice

- Stevia

Select a packet of unsweetened Kool-aid and put the contents into a blender with two cups of the sugar free soda. Then add 3cups of ice and 2½tablespoons of stevia.

To finish simply blend, pour and drink!

# 4) The Organic Slushy

You will find many shops stock an organic fruit flavor concentrate which can be used to make a natural slushy. It will be low in carbs and sugar!

Simply mix one packet of the organic fruit flavor with a teaspoon of stevia and a cup of ice. Blend to your required consistency and your slushy is ready!

This drink is refreshing even on the hottest of days!

**Ingredients**

- Orange

- Lemon

- Water

- Liquid Stevia

- Ice

Start by juicing one orange and one lemon; you must remember to remove any seeds! The juice can be added to your blender with two cups of water and 30 drops of liquid stevia. You can use the vanilla flavored stevia if you wish!

Now blend your ingredients until the mixture is smooth and taste it. You can always add more stevia to make it sweeter.

Once ready pour it into two glasses and enjoy with a friend.

# 5) The Exotic Slushy

Summer always brings images of exotic islands and lazy, sun filled days. What better way to keep the illusion alive but to enjoy a coconut slushy!

**Ingredients**

- Coconut Milk

- Coconut Water

- Stevia liquid

- Ice

As with the majority of these recipes, you will need to blend all the ingredients together. To make two slushies, mix 1 cup of coconut milk with half a cup of coconut water, a teaspoon of stevia liquid and three cups of ice.

Blend until the ice is in small particles, then pour and drink. The fresher the drink, the better the taste!

# 6) Chocolate Slushy

It is difficult to resist the chocolate slushy, especially when you realize it is possible to enjoy this delicious drink without sugar!

**Ingredients:**

- Heavy whipping cream

- Water

- Unsweetened cocoa powder

- Sugar free chocolate syrup

- Vanilla extract

Start by putting one cup of cream, ½ cup of water, 2 tablespoons of cocoa powder and ½ cup of the sugar free chocolate syrup.Slowly bring the mixture to the boil, stirring thoroughly as it does so.You can then reduce the heat to allow the mixture to simmer.At this point add in one teaspoon of vanilla and then pour it into two or three ice cube trays.

This can then be frozen for at least two hours.When you are ready to drink it simply empty the contents into your blender and pulse the mix until you reach slushy consistency.

# 7) Peach Slushy

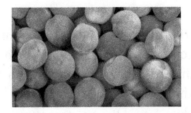

If you prefer it is possible to substitute the peaches for mangoes; or even nectarines.Both will taste just as refreshing and delicious.

**Ingredients**

- 2 peaches

- Water

- Lime juice

It is best to peel the peaches although you can leave the skin on if you prefer.To remove them you will need to pour boiling water over each peach. After thirty seconds the skin should just fall off.You will then need to remove the stones and place the peaches into your blender.

Add a teaspoon of lime juice, 50ml of water and blend.You can then consume the slushy straight away or freeze the mixture until you wish to drink it.

To add a little zing you can include 60ml of white rum or peach schnapps!

## 8) The Mango Slushy

This is another incredibly simply recipe with just a slight twist on the standard slushy option.

**Ingredients**

- Frozen Mango

- Lemon and Lime Sugar Free Soda

- Ice

Blend together a cup of frozen mango, one cup of lemon and lime soda and½cup of ice.As soon as it reaches the right consistency serve and enjoy!

## 9) Banana Slushy Surprise

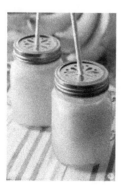

This recipe will give you a tasty, sugar free slushy with an added zing!

**Ingredients**

- 4 Bananas
- Stevia
- Water
- Pineapple juice
- Orange juice concentrate
- Lemon juice concentrate
- Ginger Ale

Unsurprisingly this slushy is made in your blender!Place the bananas a tablespoon of stevia and three cups of water into your blender and combine them.You can then add 1½cups of pineapple juice and the½cup of the orange concentrate and lemon concentrate.An additional three cups of water and blend the mixture until it is smooth.This can then be frozen until you need it; ideally split the mixture into three bottles.

When ready, add one liter of ginger ale to a bowl and one bottle of your slushy mix.Combine and enjoy your summer, sugar free punch.

# Chapter 12:10 Low Carb Cocktails

## 1) Standard Spirit & Mixer

Although not generally viewed as a cocktail, any drink which is created by mixing up liquids is a cocktail. Your standard spirit and mixer can be confidently consumed; providing you opt for the diet versions.

For example; drink gin, whiskey or rum with sugar free soda or even sparkling water. It is even possible to mix your rum with diet coke; your calorie and carb count will be zero!

## 2) Grape & Pineapple Fizz

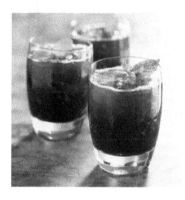

This is a refreshing and revitalizing drink at any time of the year.

**Ingredients**

- Grape juice—unsweetened
- Pineapple Juice—unsweetened

- Sugar free soda

- Ice

This is best to mix in a jug then pour as required.Mix 1½cups of grape juice with the same amount of pineapple juice.Then add in two cups of the sugar free soda and allow the mixture to chill for at least an hour.

You can garnish with mint leaves and, if desired, add a drop of your favorite liqueur.White rum is a particularly good choice!

# 3) Margarita

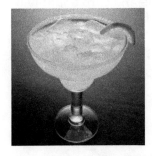

This is normally a sugar laden treat, but it can be created without the sugar input.

**Ingredients**

- Tequila

- Lime Juice

- Orange Extract

- Lime

Ideally you can mix this in a cocktail shaker, if not a jug and spoon will do!Place one shot of tequila into the shaker and add two tablespoons of lime,¼cup of water and¼teaspoon of orange extract.Shake well and pour.

To turn this into an even more refreshing drink, add ice and blend to create a slushy!

# 4) Strawberry Vodka

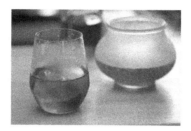

This drink will invigorate you and remind you that spring is in full flourish; with summer just round the corner!

**Ingredients**

- Vodka

- Strawberries

- Unsweetened apple juice.

- Sugar free soda water

To create this drink it is best to place several chopped strawberries into a cup of vodka and leave them overnight. You can then add half a cup of apple juice and two cups of sugar free soda water.

Mix all the ingredients together thoroughly and keep chilled. Serve over ice or even blend with ice and enjoy.

# 5) Vodka Melon

You may be surprised b y just how refreshing this delicious cocktail is!

**Ingredients**

- Watermelon
- Lime juice
- Coconut Water
- Vodka

You will need one cup of watermelon; without the seeds.You can then blend it until it is smooth and pour it into a cocktail shaker.In addition you will need to place a teaspoon of lime extract,¼cup of coconut water and½cup of vodka.

Close the shaker and make sure the ingredients are combined thoroughly.You can add some crushed ice if required.Then pour into your glasses and add a piece of lime or watermelon to garnish.

# 6) Spicy Bloody Mary

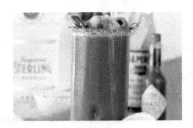

This is an ancient recipe with a small twist to add a little extra spice!

**Ingredients**

- Tomatoes
- Basil Leaves

- Pepper vodka–standard vodka can be used to reduce the'kick'
- Worcestershire sauce
- Pepper sauce

You will need to start by placing 2 cups of tomatoes into a blender with 6 basil leaves; these should be fresh.It should take a few minutes to blend them until they are smooth.The mixture can then be placed in the fridge to chill for one hour.

After the time has passed you can strain the mixture through a fine sieve; this will remove any particles.Then add it to your cocktail shaker, along with½cup of pepper vodka, 1 teaspoon of Worcestershire sauce and½teaspoon of pepper sauce.In addition some ice cubes or crushed ice can be added before you shake the mixture thoroughly.

Then simply pour it into your glass and enjoy!

# 7) Red Wine Surprise

This simple recipe adds a surprisingly tasty tang to your drink!

**Ingredients**

- Red Wine
- Sugar free (diet) ginger ale

Simple put three ounces of wine into a glass with three ounces of the ginger ale.Then stir, add an orange garnish and serve immediately.

# 8) The Mojito

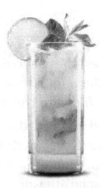

This is one drink that most people find hard to resist; it will remind you of holidays and other good times!

**Ingredients**

- Fresh Mint leaves

- Lime juice

- Vodka

- Diet soda

- Crushed ice

- Liquid stevia

The first step is to grind up the mint leaves, four or five leaves are generally enough. These should be mixed with two shots of vodka and ½ teaspoon of liquid stevia. Once this is fully mixed pour it into a glass half full of crushed ice.

Next add approximately the same amount of diet soda and, if required, a slice of lime or lemon to garnish.

# 9) Pina Colada

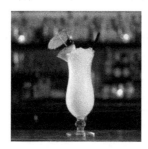

No cocktail list would be complete without a Pina Coladaand perhaps that song....

**Ingredients**

- White Rum
- Coconut Milk
- Pineapple Syrup–Must be sugar free
- Ice

Add½cup of rum to 7 tablespoons of coconut milk and 5 tablespoons of the sugar free pineapple syrup.All ingredients should be put into a blender with one cup of ice and blended for several minutes.Then drink and relax!

## 10) Mint Julep

**Ingredients**

- Bourbon
- Sugar free raspberry syrup
- Mint leaves
- Ice

Place one tablespoon of your raspberry syrup into a cup; then add several fresh mint leaves and allow them to soak up the raspberry syrup.Next, you will need to add one or two shots of bourbon; (to your own tastes) and then another tablespoon of raspberry syrup as well 1½cups of ice.

You can add a garnish if you like before you enjoy!

# Conclusion

Taking on a detox plan can seem daunting at first. However, this guide offers life-altering eating concepts and sumptuous recipes and makes the detox plan really easy to follow. With the tips, meal plans and recipes in this book, you can easily become the master of your own zero sugar diet. The book is a to-the-point, compact guide, and filled with all the necessary information you need to detox your body from sugar and overcome sugar addiction successfully.

# Part 2

# Introduction

Have you ever studied the relationship between the foods you eat and the way that you feel? Consider the way that you feel after eating a lean chicken salad for lunch vs. a fatty, carb-laden cheeseburger. If you are like most people, the cheeseburger may leave you feeling bloated and tired a few hours later. If you eat the salad, the chicken is packed full of lean protein to keep you full and nutrient-rich veggies to keep your body and mind working until your next meal.

One thing you may be thinking right now is that if eating healthy makes you feel better, why is dieting so hard? The truth is that the sugars, starches, and chemical additives in the foods found in the diets of average Americans are incredibly addictive. In fact, clinical studies evaluating the effects of sugar on the body have shown that sugar is 8 times more addictive than cocaine.

The reason why many people fail in the earlier days of diets is because they are cutting out sugars and starches (which are also loaded with sugars, even wheat products). Their body goes through withdrawal, much like it would from a drug. This results sugar cravings that make it incredibly hard to stick to a diet.

The 21-Day Sugar Detox Diet is designed to help you quickly and effectively cut sugar from your diet. As you cleanse the starches and sugars from your system, your body will not crave them anymore. You will also experience newfound health, energy, and happiness from the wholesome, nutrient-rich foods on your diet.

This book contains the information and steps you need to complete the 21-Day Sugar Detox Diet. You will learn about what foods you should cut out in the first 21 days and the foods to replace them with to help curb your carb cravings. You will also find recipes for people on the 21-Day Sugar Detox Diet, including for vegans and diabetics.

111

Thanks again for downloading this book and good luck on your future health endeavors!

# Chapter 1: An Overview Of The 21-Day Sugar Detox Diet: What It Is And How It Can Benefit You

The 21-Day Sugar Detox Diet was designed with the intention of making it easier for people to eliminate sugar from their lives. Sugars, both simple sugars and complex sugars found in carbohydrates like pasta and bread, are addictive. Think about your frequent cravings and you may find that things like candy, bread, and pasta are at the top of your list. This may be because your body is addicted to sugar. The goal of the 21-Day Sugar Detox Diet is to cleanse your body of sugar to help eliminate cravings and put you back in control.

**What's So Wrong with Sugar Anyway?**

People who are not overly conscious about the foods they eat may be surprised to learn where sugar sneaks into their diet. It is found in our drinks- from coffee to tea to soft drinks, our foods- especially fast foods and pre-packaged foods, salad dressings, condiments, bread, and many of the other foods available for a fast-paced lifestyle. In fact, the average adult eats or drinks 22 teaspoons of sugar every day. Children consume even more- 34 teaspoons every single day. Sugar is a rising epidemic, especially when you consider that nearly 25% of America's teenagers are either diabetic or in the early stages of diabetes.

The more that sugar is studied, the stronger the evidence that links it to dangerous health conditions becomes. High sugar consumption has been found to play a role in conditions like depression, dementia, certain cancers, type 2 diabetes, heart disease, male and female infertility, and even acne. Sugar also affects blood sugar levels, causing them to rise and fall at dangerous rates. If you have ever felt a mid-afternoon slump,

113

you were probably suffering from the sudden drop of your blood sugar after eating unhealthy foods for lunch.

Sugar, however, is not the only culprit of this epidemic. White and even wheat flours rise blood sugar levels quicker than sugar and these are found in almost everything that we eat. Not only do these foods raise blood sugar levels, a Harvard study found that they light up the same addiction/pleasure center of the brain as drugs like cocaine. Many others found the same results when this relationship was tested. Sugar is addictive and causes health problems and that is why you may need to detox.

**Benefits of the 21-Day Sugar Detox Diet**

The 21-Day Sugar Detox Diet offers numerous benefits. To keep things brief so we can get to the delicious recipes you can eat on the diet, here are some of the most important.

#1: Improved Energy Levels

Do you know what really causes a mid-day slump? When you eat the wrong foods, your blood sugar levels sky rocket. Not too long afterward, the food is digested and you are left feeling tired when your blood sugar plummets and craving snacks. The wholesome, nutrient-dense foods that are recommended for sugar detox stabilize your blood sugar levels and provide long-term energy. This means no more mid-day slump.

#2: Improved Weight Loss Efforts

You may or may not be trying to detox from sugar in an effort to help with weight loss. However, this is a likely result, especially if the foods you will be eating differ vastly from your typical diet. Not only will you lose weight, the fat that disappears as a result is likely to be concentrated around your belly, thighs, and butt.

#3: Better Overall Health

If you were paying attention in the previous section, you know that sugar leads to trouble for your health. The sugar detox diet will improve your long-term health and can even be used to limit medicine needed for diabetics (you should discuss the diet with your physician first). If it is followed by a lifestyle commitment to better, more wholesome eating, then you may even be able to add a few years to your life.

#4: Improved Digestion

Some of the common complaints among people following a traditional diet is gut discomfort in the form of bloating, gas, diarrhea, constipation, and other issues. Detoxing from sugar and processed foods will improve digestion and overall gut health.

#5: Clearer Skin

When you eliminate sugar and carbohydrates from your diet, you will notice clearer skin. Sugar, fat, and other ingredients in highly processed foods are known for causing hormone imbalances and skin secretions that cause acne and blackheads.

**What You Can (and Can't) Eat on the Diet**

An addiction like sugar can be handled by quitting your habit cold turkey. You cannot keep living your life according to 'just one more dinner roll and I will quit'. Carbohydrates and sugars are as addicting, if not more so, than a drug and for this reason, all sugars must be cut out of your diet completely. Part of quitting sugar knows what you can and cannot eat. While the diet will be focused around wholesome foods like proteins and nutrient-dense veggies, there are still foods that you must avoid like potatoes and similar starches. Keep reading to learn the foods to eat and avoid on the 21-Day Sugar Detox Diet.

Foods to Eat

- **Proteins-** Proteins are an essential part of the sugar detox diet, since they keep you feeling full and help balance your blood sugar. It is especially beneficial to start the morning with a breakfast packed full of protein.
- **Vegetables-** Low-starch veggies are encouraged on the 21-Day Sugar Detox Diet. They contain carbohydrates, but these are not digested the same way that starches and sugars are. In fact, you can eat as many fresh veggies as you want since they are low-calorie and full of nutrition.

Foods to Avoid

- **Processed foods**- 'Healthy' foods like yogurt and granola bars may actually be full of sugars or artificial sweeteners that harm your dieting efforts. Others like pre-made lunches and crackers are even worse. Avoid all processed foods and replace them with wholesome choices that will help curb cravings and leave you feeling full and energized.

- **Grain products**- In the first ten days of the diet, you should avoid all grain products. Switch out tortilla shells or a hamburger bun for a lettuce wrap. Avoid artificial sweeteners and additives for your coffee, as well as sports drinks and other sugar-filled products.

- **Starch-filled Vegetables**- You should also avoid any starchy vegetables in the first ten days of your diet. This includes winter squash, sweet potatoes, beats, and other potatoes (red, white, yellow, etc.).

- **Dairy**- Something else to avoid in the first 10 days of the 21-Day Sugar Detox Diet is dairy products. This is because you may have a sensitivity to the lactose in dairy without realizing it. You can switch this out for alternatives like almond milk and soy.

# Chapter 2: A Few Tips To Guide You Toward Success On The 21-Day Sugar Detox Diet

Before you check out the recipes, be sure to check out these tips. These are some guidelines that should be followed outside of the foods that you can and cannot eat to ensure success of your sugar detox.

**Tip #1: Learn How to Identify Sugars in Your Foods**

You cannot always look at the back of a food package and expect it to say 'sugar'. While some products contain just sugar, many use by-products of sugar or hide it under other names. While you are eating on the 21-day Sugar Detox Diet, you are going to remove most processed foods from your diet. If you do find yourself looking for something healthy in a hurry, though, try to avoid these sugar products and by-products:

- Sugar
- Dextrose
- Xylose
- Raw sugar
- Corn sweetener
- Evaporated cane juice
- Lactose
- Sucrose
- Evaporated cane juice
- Sugar syrup
- High-fructose corn syrup
- Fruit juice concentrates
- Agave nectar
- Beet sugar

- Fructose
- Caramel
- Rice syrup
- Corn syrup solids
- Honey
- Invert sugar
- Corn sweetener
- Malt syrup
- Cane crystals
- Barley malt
- Crystalline fructose
- Brown sugar

## #2: Choose Drinks Wisely

Even an artificial sweetener in your coffee can lead to more sugar cravings. The problem with sugary drinks is that the sugar is liquefied. Your body barely has time to break the sugar down before it flows into your liver, raises your blood sugar, and causes carb cravings that lead you to want to eat more sugar and grain products, even if you are already full.

## #3: Get Enough Sleep

Studies done on college students prove that even a few hours of sleep make a difference in sugar cravings. People who are deprived of their 8 hours of sleep crave absorbed sugars for energy. Additionally, the hormones that suppress appetite decrease and those that control hunger rise. This is a recipe for diet disaster.

## #4: Plan for Success

You have likely heard, "If you fail to plan you will plan to fail." What does it mean? It means that if you do not plan your meals, you will be more tempted to give into your unhealthy food cravings. Food prep involves making a grocery list, keeping your kitchen stocked with wholesome foods, and having prepared chicken, chopped veggies, healthy snacks, and even whole meals (ready to heat up at your convenience) on hand. It means setting aside some time early in the week to make your meals or at least prepare the ingredients so wholesome food can be on your plate in no time at all.

## #5: Always Keep Healthy Snacks on Hand

You cannot always plan when you are going to get hungry. When you are at work or running errands, you may look around and see fast foods, processed snack-machine foods, and other poor snacking choices. To keep yourself on your diet when surrounded by this temptation, keep snacks on hand. Some good options include dried veggies, granola, pumpkin seeds, nuts, turkey jerky, or unsweetened dried fruits.

# Chapter 3: Breakfast Recipes For The 21-Day Sugar Detox Diet

## Baked Cheesy Spinach Eggs

You can either use ramekins or muffin tins to make these eggs. Cook them about fifteen minutes for a 'sunny side-up' style or a little longer if you would like the yolks hard. These are great because you can throw them together, get ready for 15 minutes, and come back to a hot breakfast.

Ingredients

- 6 eggs
- 3 tablespoons olive oil
- 12 cups fresh spinach
- 1 cup low-fat mozzarella cheese (shredded)
- 2 teaspoons garlic (minced)

Instructions

Set the oven to 350 degrees so it can preheat while you prepare the eggs. Add the oil to a large skillet and add the garlic. Cook the garlic for about 1 minute, stirring frequently. Then, add the spinach to the pan and cook for 3-4 minutes. It should be wilted.

Spray six ramekins (or a 6-count muffin tin) with non-stick spray. Divide the spinach mixture evenly between these and then crack an egg over each one. Cook for 15-20 minutes, depending on how runny you want your yolks.

Add salt and pepper as desired before serving. You can eat in the ramekin (but they will be hot!) or use a knife to remove the egg onto a plate.

Nutrition Facts

Servings: 6

Calories: 160

Protein: 14 grams
Carbohydrates: 3 grams
Fat: 11 grams

# Sante-Fe Mini Frittatas

These have a slight kick of spice from the pepper jack cheese (more if you use spicy sausage) and plenty of bright veggies. These look great against the yellow background of the eggs in the muffin tin. You can top with sour cream, no sugar added salsa, fresh cilantro, or green onions if you choose.

Ingredients

- 10 eggs
- 2 egg whites
- 8 ounces pork sausage (mild or hot)
- 1 cup yellow sweet pepper (diced)
- 1 cup red sweet pepper (diced)
- ½ cup pepper jack cheese (shredded)
- ½ cup milk
- ¾ teaspoon salt
- ¼ teaspoon pepper

Instructions

Set your oven to 350 degrees so it can preheat. Cook the sausage over medium-high heat until browned. Remove the sausage with a slotted spoon and set to the side.

Add the peppers to the pan with the leftover sausage grease and saute about 3-4 minutes, until they start to soften. Set these to the side.

Take a large bowl and add the eggs, egg whites, and milk. Beat these with a whisk until well combined. Add the salt and pepper and mix to combine.

Spray a 12-count muffin tin with non-stick spray and distribute the sausage and peppers evenly. Pour the egg mixture evenly over the sausage and peppers and then top with a heaping tablespoon of pepper jack cheese. Take a fork and briefly whisk the ingredients in each muffin cup together and then cook for 25-30 minutes, until the egg is no longer runny.

Nutrition Facts
Servings: 12
Calories: 169
Protein: 11.5 grams
Carbohydrates: 3 grams
Fat: 12 grams

# Breakfast Meatballs

Meatballs for breakfast? This savory recipe has everything you would expect of a breakfast bowl, all packed into a convenient meatball. You can even prepare these ahead of time and freeze, so you only have to pull them from the freezer the night before and cook the next morning.

Ingredients

- 1 pound ground turkey
- 1 pound ground beef
- 3 large eggs
- ½ pound mild cheddar cheese (shredded)
- 2 tablespoons onion (minced)

Instructions

Start by warming the oven to 350 degrees and letting it preheat. Cover a baking sheet with aluminum foil and set to the side.

Add all the ingredients to a large mixing bowl and combine, being careful not to over mix. You can also add pepper to taste. Roll the meat mixture into balls that are 1 ½ inches in size. Cook these for 18-20 minutes, until cooked all the way through.

Nutritional Information

Servings: 8

Calories: 244

Protein: 32 grams

Carbohydrates: 1.5 grams

Fat: 11.8 grams

# Banana Pancakes

These banana pancakes should be avoided in the first week of your diet, since they do contain natural sugars from the banana. The best part is that this super simple recipe can be thrown together with just two ingredients (plus coconut oil for frying).

Ingredients

- 2 ripe bananas (there is a lower carb count if you choose a slightly less-ripe banana)
- 1 large egg
- 1 tablespoon coconut oil (for frying)

Instructions

Use a fork to mash up the bananas well. Then, add the egg and mix to combine. Warm a pan over medium-high heat and spoon the banana mixture into the pan. Allow to cook until slightly browned and firm on each side.

Nutritional Facts

Servings: 2

Calories: 195

Protein: 4.5 grams

Carbohydrates: 23 grams

Fat: 10 grams

# Chapter 4: Main Course Recipes For The 21-Day Sugar Detox Diet

## Lemon Garlic Chicken Drumsticks

Bright lemon and savory garlic come together in this recipe. As an added benefit, you can use leftover chicken to make a salad the next day. You could also use chicken thighs or breasts, though these may need longer to cook. Always make sure you cook your chicken through to prevent the risk of salmonella and other foodborne illness.

Ingredients

- 8 chicken drumsticks
- 3 garlic cloves (minced)
- ¼ cup fresh parsley (chopped)
- 3 tablespoons lemon juice (the juice of about 2 lemons)
- Zest of 1 lemon
- 1 teaspoon dried Italian seasoning
- 2 tablespoons butter
- 2 tablespoons olive oil
- 1 teaspoon salt
- 1 teaspoon pepper

Instructions

Add the olive oil to a saute pan over medium high heat. Mix together the salt, pepper, and Italian seasoning in a small bowl and stir with a fork until combined.

Top the chicken drumsticks with the seasoning and add them to the pan. Sear on each side until they are browned, about 1-2 minutes per side. Then, cover the pan with a lid and turn down to a simmer for about 20 minutes.

Place the drumsticks on a plate and try to keep them warm. Then, turn the pan to low heat and add the butter and garlic. Stir together for 1-2 minutes until very fragrant. Then, add the lemon juice and zest to the pan. Mix together and return the drumsticks to the pan. Spoon the lemon-garlic-butter sauce over the chicken and top with fresh parsley before serving.

Nutrition Facts

Servings: 8

Calories: 154

Protein: 14 grams

Carbohydrates: > 0.5 grams

Fat: 10.5 grams

# Meatloaf

This savory meatloaf is low-carb. It makes a great main course addition to a flavorful salad, cauliflower mash, or a side of soup. It can also easily be reheated for lunch the next day.

Ingredients

- 2 pounds ground beef
- 1 cup homemade broth
- 1/3 cup tomato paste
- 1 medium onion (diced)
- 1 red pepper (diced)
- 1 green pepper (diced)
- 1 garlic clove (minced)
- 1 tablespoon coconut oil
- 1 tablespoon cumin
- 1 teaspoon paprika

Instructions

Start by setting the oven to 350 degrees so it can preheat. Line a rimmed baking tray with parchment paper and set aside.

Add the coconut oil to a skillet and warm over medium heat. Add the diced peppers and onions to the pan and sprinkle salt and pepper across the top. Saute for 3 minutes and then add the garlic. Continue to cook an additional minute or two, until the garlic is fragrant and becoming translucent.

Transfer the onion and pepper mixture to a large bowl and add the meat and spices. Mix them until well combined, but be careful not to over mix.

Form a loaf with your mixture, making it square-shaped to fit the baking tray. It should be about three inches thick. Set this to the side.

Take the pan that you prepared the vegetable mixture in and add the broth and tomato paste. Warm these over medium heat until you bring to a simmer. Simmer for 7-10 minutes, until the mixture thickens. Spread this on top of the meatloaf you set aside and put in the oven for about 45 minutes, or until the meat is cooked all the way through.

Nutrition Facts

Servings: 6

Calories: 342

Protein: 48.5 grams

Carbohydrates: 8.5 grams

Fat: 12.5 grams

# Broccoli Mushroom Chicken Casserole

This dish is packed full of protein-rich chicken, nutrient-rich broccoli, and hearty mushrooms. Even though this dish is packed with flavor, you can top with cheese and broil for a minute before serving if you would like.

Ingredients

- 3 cups cooked chicken (shredded)
- 1 cup low-sodium chicken broth
- 4 cups fresh broccoli florets (cleaned and chopped)
- 1 cup Portobello mushrooms (cleaned and sliced)
- 1 medium onion (diced)
- 2 eggs
- 1 cup full-fat coconut milk
- 1 tablespoon + 1 tablespoon coconut oil (divided)
- ½ teaspoon nutmeg
- Sea salt and pepper

Instructions

Start by setting the oven to 350 degrees to preheat. Use 1 tablespoon of the coconut oil and grease a 9x13 casserole dish. Set to the side.

Steam the broccoli 10-15 minutes, until barely cooked. Set this to the side.

Add the coconut oil to a saucepan and warm over medium high heat. Brown the onions for 3-4 minutes and sprinkle salt and pepper over them. Add the mushrooms to the pan and stir, cooking for about 4-5 minutes until tender. Stir in the cooked chicken and broccoli until combined and layer it across the bottom of the prepared casserole dish.

In a medium bowl, add the chicken broth, eggs, coconut milk, nutmeg, and sea salt and pepper to taste. Whisk these until well combined and then pour over the casserole dish so the chicken broccoli mixture is covered. Cook for 35-40 minutes, until the casserole begins to firm up. Allow to sit for at least ten minutes before cutting.

Nutrition Facts

Servings: 4

Calories: 312

Protein: 39 grams

Carbohydrates: 11 grams

Fat: 13 grams

# Garlic Dijon Salmon

Spicy Dijon and flavorful garlic come together beautifully with tender, flaky salmon. This can be served on top of a salad or alongside any of your favorite side dishes.

Ingredients

- 4 salmon fillets with skin (about 6 ounces each)
- 1 red onion (thinly sliced)
- 4 large garlic cloves (thinly sliced)
- 1/3 cup Dijon mustard
- 1 teaspoon tarragon (dried)
- Salt and pepper to taste

Instructions

Start by setting the oven to 400 degrees. Coat a 9x13 baking pan with cooking spray. Then, set the salmon with the skin down on the baking pan. Coat the top with Dijon mustard and sprinkle the onion and garlic slices on top. Sprinkle the tarragon and salt and pepper on the top.

Allow the salmon to cook for 20 minutes, until it is warmed through and flaky. Serve with your choice of side.

Nutritional Facts

Servings: 4

Calories: 305

Protein: 30 grams

Carbohydrates: 8.5 grams

Fat: 16 grams

# Chicken Cordon Bleu

This recipe is packed full of protein. While it is high in fat and calories, it has less than 10 carbs. It is a savory dish that can be enjoyed by anyone on the 21-Day Sugar Detox Diet. Make sure you have toothpicks handy, as these will stop your chicken rolls from unrolling.

Ingredients

- 6 chicken breast halves (boneless, skinless)
- 6 slices ham
- 6 slices Swiss cheese
- ½ cup dry white wine
- 1 teaspoon chicken bouillon granules
- 3 tablespoons all-purpose flour
- 6 tablespoons butter
- 1 cup heavy whipping cream
- 1 tablespoon cornstarch

Instructions

Your chicken breasts need to be thin enough that you can roll them. If they are not, use a meat tenderizer to pound them until they are thin enough. In each breast, place one slice of ham and one slice of Swiss cheese. Position them about ½ an inch from one side. Fold over starting at the side nearest to the ham and cheese, rolling to the end of the chicken and then securing with a toothpick. Once your roll-ups are finished, place these off to the side.

Add the flour and paprika to a small bowl and use a fork to stir. Set this to the side while you prepare the pan for cooking.

Heat the butter to a medium-high heat in a large skillet. Sear the chicken on all sides, browning them slightly. Add the bouillon cube and the wine and reduce the heat to a simmer. Cover the chicken and cook for about 30 minutes, until cooked all the way through.

Once cooked, remove the chicken and place on a warmed plate. Set this to the side while you add the cornstarch and heavy cream to a small bowl. Whisk this into the wine mixture in the skillet and stir until it becomes thick and gravy-like. Pour this over the chicken and serve.

Nutritional Facts

Servings: 6

Calories: 580

Protein: 41 grams

Carbohydrates: 8 grams

Fat: 41 grams

# Grilled Shrimp

This grilling recipe requires you to marinate the shrimp beforehand. Even though it calls for a little cayenne paper, you cannot even taste it. This means that if you can convince your kids to put one of these curly guys in their mouth, they will love its sweet and smoky flavor as much as you do. You will need skewers to prepare these shrimp.

Ingredients

- 2 pounds fresh shrimp (peeled and deveined)
- ¼ cup tomato sauce
- 3 garlic cloves (minced)
- 2 tablespoons fresh basil (chopped)
- 1/3 cup olive oil
- 2 tablespoons red wine vinegar
- ¼ teaspoon cayenne pepper
- ½ teaspoon salt

Instructions

Add the tomato sauce, olive oil, vinegar, and garlic in a large bowl and use a whisk to mix until well combined. Then, add the basil, cayenne pepper, and salt and mix again. Finally, add the shrimp to the mixture and stir until well coated.

Cover the bowl with the shrimp and let it marinate in the refrigerator for at least one hour. You will want to stir every 20 minutes or so, to ensure the shrimp marinates evenly.

When you are ready to cook, set the grill to medium heat while you prepare the shrimp. Insert skewers through a few shrimp, being sure not to pack them too tightly so they can cook all the way through. The best way to keep them on the skewers is by piercing once through the head and once through the tail.

When the shrimp skewers are ready and the grill is preheated, brush oil onto the grill grate to prevent the shrimp from sticking.

Put the kabobs on the grill and cook for 2-3 minutes on each side, until lightly charred and opaque.

Nutritional Facts

Servings: 6

Calories: 275

Protein: 31 grams

Carbohydrates: 3 grams

Fat: 14.5 grams

# Garlic-Y Prime Rib

This prime rib is marinated beforehand. This lets it be cook in under 2 hours, though it tastes like it simmered away all day. The garlic also sinks deep down into the prime rib, flavoring the entire cut of meat.

Ingredients

- 3 pounds prime rib roast
- 4 garlic cloves (minced)
- 2 teaspoons dried thyme
- 2 tablespoons olive oil
- 2 teaspoons salt
- 2 teaspoon black pepper

Instructions

Take a roasting pan and place the roast inside, leaving the fatty side facing up. Set this aside as you mix the olive oil, garlic, and spices together in a bowl. Spread this mixture on the roast and let it sit out until it reaches room temperature, usually 30-45 minutes. Be caution not to let the roast warm too much.

Preheat the oven to 500 degrees. Once it is ready, put the prime rib inside and cook for 15 minutes. Turn down the temperature so it is 325 degree and cook for an additional 45-60 minutes. Use a meat thermometer to prevent overcooking. For a medium rare roast, you want an internal temperature of 135 degrees.

Once you remove the roast from the oven, do not cut into it right away. Allow it to sit and retain its juices for at least 10 minutes before cutting and serving.

Nutritional Facts

Servings: 6

Calories: 190

Protein: 13 grams

Carbohydrates: 0.8 grams

Fat: 19 grams

# Chapter 5: Side Dish Recipes For The 21-Day Sugar Detox Diet

## Fresh Zucchini Noodles

These zucchini 'noodles' are the perfect companion for chicken, seafood, or pork chops, as well as served as a side topped with feta cheese, almonds, dried fruit, or other ingredients. The best part is there are no 'noodles' in here. The only carbohydrates from this come from the natural fiber and sugar in zucchini.

Ingredients

- 6 cups (about 4 medium) zucchini
- 2 tablespoons fresh parsley (chopped)
- 2 tablespoons fresh basil (chopped)
- 3 tablespoons lemon juice
- 3 tablespoons olive oil
- ½ teaspoon salt
- ¼ teaspoon pepper

Instructions

Grate, slice, or shred your zucchini into a large bowl and set to the side. In a small bowl, whisk together the olive oil, lemon juice, herbs, salt, and pepper. Pour this over the zucchini and toss.

Nutrition Facts

Servings: 6

Calories: 83

Protein: 2 grams

Carbohydrates: 5 grams

Fat: 7 grams

# Cooked 'Zoodles'

Like the previous recipe, these zucchini noodles are low-carb. These are gently cooked so they are warm though, making them the perfect companion for chicken alfredo, spaghetti, and other dishes where you want to replace noodles.

Ingredients

- 5-6 large zucchini
- ¼ cup olive oil
- 1 cup water
- ½ teaspoon salt
- ¼ teaspoon pepper

Instructions

You can leave the skin on the zucchini or peel it, depending on how 'noodle-like' you want your zoodles to be. Peel the zucchini into long strips with a vegetable peeler (or use a mandolin). Discard the zucchini seeds and the cut the peels you made into long strips so they resemble the thickness of spaghetti.

Add the olive oil to a large skillet and warm over medium heat. Once heated, add the zucchini and stir it around. Cook for 1 minute and then add the water, salt, and pepper. Allow to cook until the zucchini starts to become soft, but watch it closely so it does not become mushy. This should take 5-7 minutes.

Nutrition Facts

Servings: 4

Calories: 157

Protein: 3 grams

Carbohydrates: 8 grams

Fat: 14 grams

# Cheesy 'Bread' Sticks

Cauliflower is the secret ingredient in this delicious recipe. These sticks taste great with your choice of marinara sauce (no-sugar added, of course). You should cut them into shorter pieces than you typically would with bread sticks, since they are a little flimsier. You'll be delighted to know that they are just as crisp, though!

Ingredients

- 1 head cauliflower
- 2 egg whites
- 1 cup mozzarella cheese (shredded)
- 1 cup Parmesan cheese (grated)
- 1 teaspoon garlic powder
- 1 teaspoon Italian seasoning
- ½ teaspoon salt

Instructions

Start by setting the oven to 450 to preheat. Prepare the cauliflower by washing it and drying it. You should have about 4 cups once it is chopped. Set the dried cauliflower to the side.

Take parchment paper and layer it across 2 8x12 baking sheets. Roughly chop the cauliflower into bite-sized pieces. Either microwave for 7-8 minutes or steam the cauliflower for 20. Once cooked, allow to cool for a few minutes and add to the food processor. Pulse the cauliflower until it looks like pieces of rice.

Add the pulsed cauliflower to a large bowl and add all the ingredients except the mozzarella cheese. Spread this across the baking sheets and cook for 30 minutes, until it is brown across the top. Then, sprinkle the mozzarella cheese on the baked cauliflower mixture and pop it in the broiler for one minute, until the cheese is melted. Allow this to rest at least 10 minutes before slicing it into 24 pieces.

Nutrition Facts

Servings: 4
Calories: 189
Protein: 18 grams
Carbohydrates: 5 grams
Fat: 11 grams

# Turkey 'Noodle' Soup

This hearty dish is perfect after Thanksgiving, especially since it calls for turkey broth that you can easily make from your leftover turkey carcass. The 'noodles' are made of spaghetti squash, which is a filling additive to this hearty soup.

Ingredients

- 3 cups baked spaghetti squash
- 6 cups homemade turkey broth
- 3 cups cooked turkey (shredded)
- 1 medium onion (diced)
- 2 carrots (sliced)
- 3 celery stalks (diced)
- 1 tablespoon butter or coconut oil
- ¼ fresh parsley (chopped)
- Sea salt and pepper to taste

Instructions

Prepare the spaghetti squash by cutting it in half and brushing it with olive oil. Sprinkle salt and pepper across the top of it and place the squash with the skin side down on a baking tray. Bake for about 50-90 minutes at 375 degrees, until the squash is tender.

Melt the butter in the bottom of a soup pot and add the carrots, celery, and onions. Sprinkle with the salt and pepper and stir. Cook over medium heat for 5 minutes. Then, add the turkey, broth, and parsley. Bring this to a simmer and allow to cook for 20 minutes.

Use a fork to pull apart the spaghetti squash into noodle-like strings. Add these to the pot on the stove and cook an additional ten minutes.

*Note: To make turkey broth, start by roasting your turkey bones in the oven at 350 degrees for 20 minutes. Add these to a large pot on the stove with chopped carrots and celery, sea salt, herbs, and whatever spices you would like your broth to be flavored with. Allow this to cook on low heat for 12-24 hours. Alternatively, you could make your broth on low heat in the crock pot. You can use this method for almost any type of homemade broth.

Nutrition Facts

Servings: 4

Calories: 270

Protein: 35 grams

Carbohydrates: 13 grams

Fat: 8.5 grams

# Smothered Green Beans

Bacon, minced onions, and green beans cooked so they are juicy but still have a snap come together in this dish. It makes eating your vegetables fun and the bacon adds a little protein you wouldn't normally get from your vegetable side dish.

Ingredients

- 1 pound fresh green beans
- 6 slices thick bacon (chopped)
- 1 medium onion (minced)
- 2 garlic cloves (minced)
- 1 cup water
- Salt and pepper to taste

Instructions

Start by preparing your green beans. Wash them and trim off all the ends. Set to the side.

Choose a skillet deep enough to cook your green beans. Bring to temperature over medium high heat and add your chopped bacon. Once the fat starts to render from the bacon, stir in the garlic and onions. Cook for one minute before you add the water and green beans.

Continue cooking over medium high heat until the water evaporates. Check the green beans. If they are not tender enough, add a little more water. Season with salt and pepper to your preference just before serving.

Nutritional Facts

Servings: 6

Calories: 100

Protein: 6.5 grams

Carbohydrates: 7 grams

Fat: 5.5 grams

# Prosciutto Wrapped Asparagus

This is a side dish packed with flavor and light on the carbs. It has added protein from the prosciutto, as well as a great salty flavor that pairs well with asparagus. It is so fancy it can dress up almost any dish.

Ingredients

- 12 fresh spears asparagus (trimmed)
- 4 ounces reduced-fat cream cheese (softened)
- ½ pound prosciutto (sliced)

Instructions

Start by setting the oven to 450 degrees so it can preheat while you are preparing the asparagus. Gently coat a baking sheet with non-stick spray and set to the side.

Spread the softened cream cheese on the prosciutto slices. Stick a bunch of 2-3 asparagus spears and roll up. Arrange these with the folded side down on the prepared baking sheet. Cook for approximately 15 minutes, until the asparagus becomes tender.

Nutritional Facts

Servings: 4

Calories: 292

Protein: 14.6 grams

Carbohydrates: 2.7 grams

Fat: 25 grams

# Creamy Cucumber Salad

This cool, creamy salad is satisfying as a side dish. It pairs well with grilled chicken or fish, or even a hamburger. You can eat this the way the recipe suggests, or you can add sliced onions and plump, juicy tomatoes for a twist.

Ingredients

- 1 large cucumber (cleaned and sliced)
- 1 cup mayonnaise
- ¼ cup milk
- ½ teaspoon white vinegar
- ¼ teaspoon garlic powder
- ¼ teaspoon onion powder
- Salt and pepper to taste

Instructions

Add the mayonnaise, milk, and vinegar to a medium-sized bowl and whisk until the mixture is smooth. Then, stir in the onion and garlic powder. Mix to combine and stir in the cucumbers, coating evenly. Allow the cucumber salad to chill in the refrigerator for at least 30 minutes. You can stir in salt and pepper just before you serve or you can serve to the side so people can salt and pepper to their taste.

Nutritional Facts

Servings: 4

Calories: 410

Protein: 1.5 grams

Carbohydrates: 6 grams

Fat: 42 grams

# Chapter 6: Snack And Dessert Recipes For The 21-Day Detox Diet

## Mini Zucchini Cheese Bites

You can eat four of these delightful bites for just over 4 carbohydrates and under 100 calories. They are crispy and cheesy- the perfect snack when you are craving chips or cheez-its.

Ingredients

- 2 cups zucchini (about 2 large zucchini)
- 1 egg
- ¼ cup cilantro (this can be omitted if you do not like cilantro)
- ½ cup Parmesan cheese (grated)
- ½ teaspoon salt
- ¼ teaspoon pepper

Instructions

Set the oven to 400 degrees to preheat. Spray a 12-count mini muffin tin with non-stick spray and set to the side.

Roughly cut the zucchini into chunks and grate it in your food processor. Place in cheesecloth or several paper towels and squeeze out the extra liquid. Add this to a bowl and mix in all the other ingredients.

Divide this into the 12 muffin cups and press down firmly, packing the mixture down. Bake 15 minutes or longer, until the edges of the zucchini cup turn golden brown.

Nutrition Facts

Servings: 3

Calories: 97

Protein: 8.6 grams

Carbohydrates: 4.3 grams

**Fat: 5.3 grams**

# Spicy Mediterranean Dip

This dip makes for a great low-carb dip for cucumbers, celery, carrots, zucchini sticks, broccoli, or any other veggies you want. It is creamy but also has a kick, though you can adjust the amount of Tabasco sauce if you do not like spicy. This dip also has a nice crunch (and added protein) from walnuts.

Ingredients

- 1 cup reduced fat feta cheese (crumbled)
- ¼ cup toasted walnuts (you can toast these in the oven if you cannot find them toasted)
- ¼ cup unsweetened almond milk
- ¼ cup nonfat Greek yogurt (plain)
- ¼ cup roasted red peppers (chopped)
- Juice of 1 lemon (about 1 ½ tablespoons)
- 2 teaspoons extra virgin olive oil
- ¼ teaspoon Tabasco sauce
- ¼ teaspoon pepper

Instructions

Add all the ingredients to a food processor (you can use a blender if you do not have a food processor that is large enough). Pulse them together until the dip is your desired consistency. Refrigerate until you are ready to eat.

Nutrition Facts

Servings: 8

Calories: 90

Protein: 5 grams

Carbohydrates: 2.5 grams

Fat: 6.7 grams

# Low-Carb Sushi

This makes for a great snack (or double-up and use it for lunch). It has plenty of sushi flavors but is easy to make. You can serve with a bottle of Coconut Aminos.

Ingredients

- 1 package Seaweed wrappers
- 6 ounces tuna
- 2 medium avocados (peeled, pitted, and thinly sliced)
- 1 large carrot (shredded)
- 1 cup cilantro leaves (chopped)
- ¼ cup kimchi (optional)
- 1 cucumber (thinly sliced)
- 1 bunch green onions (cleaned and sliced)

Instructions

Place the seaweed wrapper on a plate and assemble the ingredients into a 1-inch wide section of the wrap. Use a small bowl of water to wet your finger and run it along the very edge of the wrap, on the opposite side of your filling. Then, starting at the end with the ingredients, roll the seaweed wrapper. Try to keep it as tight as you can and be sure not to overfill. This may take some practice, but you will be rolling like a pro in no time at all.

Nutrition Facts

Servings: 2

Calories: 215

Protein: 25 grams

Carbohydrates: 9.5 grams

Fat: 7 grams

# Pumpkin Custard

This is a savory pumpkin recipe since there is no added sweetener. If you are in the later days of the diet, you can add your choice of sweetener so this recipe satisfies your sweet tooth.

Ingredients

- 1 cup canned full-fat coconut milk
- 1 cup canned pumpkin
- 2 eggs
- 1 teaspoon vanilla extract
- 2 teaspoon cinnamon
- ¼ teaspoon grated nutmeg
- ¼ teaspoon ground ginger

Instructions

Start by setting the oven to 350 degrees to preheat. Add the pumpkin and spices in a medium sized bowl. In a small bowl, use a whisk to gently beat the eggs and then whisk in the coconut milk and vanilla. Once combined, mix this into the bowl of spiced pumpkin mixture and stir until combined.

You can prepare this in a medium-sized ceramic baking dish or 6 ramekins that are ½ cup in size each. Take a deep baking pan and place either the dish or the ramekins on the tray. Add water until it reaches 2" up the side of your baking dish. Cook for about an hour, or until you can insert a fork or knife into the center of the pumpkin custard and pull it out clean.

Nutrition Facts

Servings: 3

Calories: 118

Protein: 7 grams

Carbohydrates: 11.5 grams

Fat: 5 grams

# Kale Chips

Kale is packed full of vitamins and nutrients. When prepared this way, it is crunchy, salty, and everything else you need to satisfy a potato chip craving. Also, when you make this recipe at home you save a lot of money compared to buying high-end kale chips from the health food store.

Ingredients

- 6 cups kale (about 2-3 bunches)
- 2 tablespoons coconut oil
- Sea salt and your choice of seasonings

Instructions

Start by setting the oven to 350 degrees and allowing to preheat. While you are waiting, clean your kale and chop it into bite size pieces. Dab with paper towels or use a salad spinner to get it dry.

Then, take a baking sheet and spread the kale across it. Break the coconut oil up into pieces and place it on top of the kale. Sprinkle your seasonings on top of this and roast for 10 minutes. You can leave it in longer for a crispier kale chip.

Nutritional Information

Servings: 2

Calories: 108

Protein: 4 grams

Carbohydrates: 9 grams

Fat: 6.4 grams

# Baked Cinnamon Apples Topped With Almonds

Warm, tender apples, spicy cinnamon, and crunchy almonds come together in this dessert. This will satisfy your sweet tooth without leaving you regretting it later.

Ingredients

- 2 large Granny Smith apples
- ¾ cup sliced almonds
- 2 teaspoons cinnamon
- ½ teaspoon ground clove
- 1 tablespoon coconut oil

Instructions

Set the oven to 350 degrees so it can preheat. Peel and core the apples. Then, dice them into bite-sized pieces. Add these to a medium-sized bowl and add the other ingredients, stirring to combine. Distribute this into 4 muffin cup holders or 4 ramekins and bake for 20 minutes.

Nutritional Information

Servings: 4

Calories: 102

Protein: 6 grams

Carbohydrates: 15 grams

Fat: 3.5 grams

# Pepperoni Pizza Bites

These have the consistency of tater tots and the flavor of pepperoni pizza, but without all the processed ingredients and carbohydrates. They are also pretty filling, since the base is made of cauliflower and they have a good protein punch. They taste great served with marinara or another dipping sauce.

Ingredients

- 2 pounds cauliflower florets (cleaned)
- 6 cups water
- 2 large eggs
- 8 slices pepperoni (diced)
- 1/3 cup coconut flour
- 1 tablespoon Italian seasoning
- ½ teaspoon garlic powder
- ½ teaspoon salt

Instructions

Start by preheating the oven to 350 degrees. Then, bring the water to boil in a large pan and then add the cauliflower florets. Boil for about 4 minutes and drain. Once the cauliflower has cooled completely, dice it. You should note that you should not use a food processor, since it will make the cauliflower too small.

Add the cauliflower to a large bowl with the diced pepperoni, coconut flour, and spices. Mix to combine before adding the eggs and stirring until well-combined. Set this to the side.

Line a baking sheet with parchment paper. Take the cauliflower-pepperoni mixture and make tater tot-shaped bites. Cook for 45-50 minutes, until the tots are golden brown in color and crispy on the outside.

Nutritional Facts

Servings: 8

Calories: 86

Protein: 5.3 grams

Carbohydrates: 6.4 grams
Fat: 4.5 grams

# Sugar Busters Diet Recipes And Meal Plan

## Easy And Delicious Breakfast Recipes
## Avocado Coconut Green Smoothie

Preparation Time: 5 Minutes

Cooking Time: N/A

Serves: 2

Ingredients:

- 1 to 1 ½ cups unsweetened almond milk
- ¼ cup freshly grated coconut meat
- 1 ½ cups diced fresh avocado, frozen if desired
- 2 cups loosely packed kale
- 1/3 cup of protein powder


- 1 to 2 packets of stevia, or as needed to taste

**Directions:**

1.Mix together all ingredients in a high speed blender, turn to medium-low speed and pulse for about 30 seconds.

2.Adjust to high speed and pulse until thick and smooth. Portion green smoothie into two serving glasses and serve immediately.

# Mixed Berry Coconut Smoothie

Preparation Time: 5 Minutes

Cooking Time: N/A

Serves: 2

Ingredients:
- 2 scoops of vegan protein powder
- 1 cup frozen blueberries
- 1 cup fresh raspberries
- ½ cup fresh blackberries
- ½ cup fresh or unsweetened coconut milk

- ¾ to 1 cup of coconut water

**Directions:**

1.Combine all ingredients in a high speed blender or food processor and pulse for about 30 to 45 seconds on medium-low speed. Adjust to high speed and pulse until thick and smooth.

2.Portion into individual serving glasses and serve immediately.

# Coconut Flour Waffles

Preparation time: 10 minutes

Cooking time: 10 minutes

Serves: 4

Ingredients:

- ¼ cup of vegan or grass-fed butter
- 4 large free range fresh eggs
- 1 small pinch of real salt
- ½ teaspoon of baking powder
- 5 tablespoons of sifted coconut flour
- 1 to 1 ½ packets of stevia powder


- Olive oil or grass-fed ghee, for greasing

**Directions:**

1.Place the butter and eggs in a mixing bowl and whisk thoroughly until smooth and creamy. Set aside.

2.In a separate bowl, add the rest of the ingredients and mix until well combined. Gradually add the dry mixture into the bowl with the butter-egg mixture while mixing constantly until smooth and well incorporated. Cover the bowl with cloth or plastic wrap and let it rest for about 10 minutes.

3.Preheat the waffle maker and lightly brush the grid with ghee or oil. Once the waffle iron is hot, pour with enough batter and cook according to the recommended cooking time by waffle maker. Remove the cooked waffle, transfer to a plate and repeat procedure with remaining batter.

4.Serve warm with your favorite toppings, if desired.

# Blueberry Almond Pancakes

Preparation time: 10 minutes

Cooking time: 15 to 20 minutes

Serves: 4 to 6

Ingredients:

- 4 large free range fresh eggs
- ¼ cup of warm water
- ¼ cup of unsweetened almond milk
- ¼ cup softened grass-fed or vegan butter
- 2 cups of sifted almond flour
- 1 teaspoon of baking soda
- ½ teaspoon of real salt
- 2 packets of stevia powder
- ½ cup fresh blueberries

- Grass-fed ghee or olive oil, for greasing

**Directions:**

1.In a large mixing bowl, mix together all wet ingredients and whisk until smooth and well combined.

2.Add all dry ingredients in a high speed blender, mix in the wet mixture and pulse until the mixture is smooth and well incorporated. Return into the bowl and fold in the blueberries. Cover with plastic wrap and let it stand for about 5 to 10 minutes before cooking.

3.Lightly grease a medium pan and apply with medium-high heat. Once the skillet is hot, pour with enough batter or about ½ cup just to cover the bottom of the pan. Swirl to evenly coat the bottom of the pan and cook for about 2 to 3 minutes on each side, or until lightly golden. Flip to cook the other side and repeat procedure with the remaining batter.

4.Transfer into individual serving plates and top with cubed butter, if desired. Serve immediately.

# Spinach And Tomato Omelette

Preparation time: 5 minutes

Cooking time: 5 minutes

Serves: 3 to 4

Ingredients:

- 4 large free-range fresh eggs, lightly beaten
- ¼ cup diced shallots
- 1 cup loosely packed fresh baby spinach
- ½ cup quartered cherry tomatoes
- ¼ cup grated nonfat Swiss cheese


- 2 to 3 teaspoons of olive oil

**Directions:**

1.Add the oil in a medium skillet or pan and apply with medium-high heat. Add in the shallots and tomatoes and sauté for about 2 to 3 minutes, or until soft and tender.

2.Spread the sautéed vegetables on the bottom of the skillet and pour in the beaten eggs.

3.Place the spinach and the cheese on one side of the egg mixture and reduce heat to medium-low. Carefully lift the side without the toppings and fold to cover the spinach and cheese.

4.Cook until the bottom is lightly golden and turn to cook the other side for 1 to 2 minutes, or until the omelette is cooked through. Remove from heat and slide the omelette on a serving plate.

5.Slice the omellete into 2 equal portions and serve immediately.

# Cucumber Salad With Fried Hemp Tofu

Preparation time: 10 minutes

Cooking time: 10 minutes

Serves: 4

**Ingredients:**

For the Salad:

- 2 large cucumber, sliced into thin rounds
- 1 large red onion, halved and thinly sliced
- 1 ripe red tomato, seeded and sliced into thin rounds

- Crushed red pepper flakes, real salt and black pepper

For the Hemp Fu:

- 8 ounces of firm hemp or soy tofu, pressed and drained, cut into thin slices
- 1 tablespoon of extra virgin olive oil

- 1 teaspoon of mixed Italian herbs

For the Dressing:

- ½ teaspoon minced garlic
- 1 tablespoon soy sauce (namu shoyu or coconut aminos)
- 1 teaspoons apple cider vinegar
- ½ cup of olive oil
- ½ teaspoon of toasted sesame oil

- Real salt and ground black pepper, to taste

**Directions:**

1.Season sliced tofu with Italian herbs, salt and black pepper and rub evenly on all sides. Set aside.

2.In a large skillet, apply medium-high heat and add the oil. When the oil is hot, fry the tofu in separate batches for about 4 minutes on each side or until lightly browned. Turn to cook the other side for about 3 to 4 minutes, or until lightly golden. Transfer to a plate lined with paper towels, cook the remaining batch and set aside to drain excess oil.

3.While cooking the hemp tofu, mix together all dressing ingredients in a small bowl and whisk until well combined. Set aside.

4.In a serving bowl, combine all salad ingredients and pour in the dressing. Gently toss to evenly coat the cucumber with salad dressing, season to taste with salt and pepper and top with fried tofu. Sprinkle with red pepper flakes on top and serve immediately.

# Zucchini Breakfast Patties

Preparation time: 20 minutes

Cooking time: 15 minutes

Serves: 8

Ingredients:

· 1 pound raw zucchini, julienned or spiralized

· 3 large organic free-range eggs

· ¼ cup diced shallots

· 1 teaspoon of mixed Italian herbs

· ½ cup almond meal or flour

· ¼ cup of unsweetened desiccated coconut

· Fleur de sel and black pepper, to taste

· 1 ½ tablespoons olive oil

**Directions:**

1.In a large mixing bowl, add the zucchini and sprinkle with ¼ teaspoon of salt. Gently toss to combine and transfer to a colander. Let it stand for about 30 to 45 minutes to drain excess water and squeeze to remove the remaining moisture.

2.While draining the zucchini, combine together eggs, Italian herbs, almond meal, desiccated coconut and a pinch of salt and pepper in a separate mixing bowl. Mix until well combined, stir in the drained zucchini and chill for at least 15 to 20 minutes.

3.Divide the zucchini mixture into 8 equal portions and form each into a ball. Place it on a baking sheet lined with parchment paper and lightly press down to from them into patties.

4.In a large nonstick skillet, apply medium-high heat and add in half of the oil. When the oil hot, fry the zucchini patties in separate batches for about 5 to 6 minutes on each side or until lightly browned. Turn to cook the other side, remove from the skillet and transfer to a plate lined with paper towels.

5.Add in the rest of the oil and repeat cooking procedure with the remaining patties. Remove from heat, place it on the plate with paper towels and set aside for a about 5 minutes to drain excess oil.

6.Transfer into a serving platter and serve immediately.

# Healthy, Filling Lunch Recipes
## Kale And Broccoli Egg White Quiche

Preparation time: 10 minutes

Cooking time: 50 minutes

Serves: 4

Ingredients:
- 1 cup packed fresh kale
- 1 cup detached broccoli florets
- 2 cups of free range egg whites, lightly beaten
- 1 medium onion, thinly sliced
- 1 large red sweet pepper, seeded and sliced into thin strips
- ¼ teaspoon onion powder
- ½ teaspoon mixed Italian herbs
- Real salt and black pepper, to taste
- 2 tablespoons of grass fed ghee or olive oil, for greasing

- ½ teaspoon of minced fresh parsley, for serving

**Directions:**

1.Preheat an oven to 375°F, lightly grease a pie dish with ghee or oil and set aside.

2.In a large skillet or sauté pan, apply with medium-high heat and add in the remaining ghee or oil. Add the onion and pepper and sauté until soft and tender. Stir in the broccoli, cook until soft while stirring occasionally and add in the kale. Season with Italian herbs, garlic powder, salt and black pepper and cook until the kale is lightly wilted.

3.Remove from heat, transfer into the prepared pie dish and pour in the beaten egg whites. Briefly stir ingredients and evenly spread on the bottom of the pie dish.

4.Bake it in the oven for about 30 to 35 minutes, or until the center is set and quiche is cooked through. Remove from the oven and let it stand for about 5 to 10 minutes.

5.Slice into 4 equal portions and transfer into individual serving plates. Serve immediately with parsley on top.

6.Bake it in the oven for about 35 to 40 minutes, or until the center is set. Remove it from the oven and let it rest for about 5 minutes before serving.

# Spinach And Mushroom Frittata

Preparation time: 15 minutes

Cooking time: 45 minutes

Serves: 4 to 6

Ingredients:

- 1 cup diced fresh portabella mushroom
- 1 cup packed fresh kale
- 1 teaspoon minced garlic
- 1 tablespoon minced shallot
- 4 large free range whole eggs
- ½ cup almond milk
- 1 teaspoon mixed Italian herbs
- Real salt and ground black pepper, to taste

- Olive oil or grass fed ghee, for greasing

**Directions:**

1.Preheat an oven to 350°F and lightly grease a pie dish and set aside.

2.In a skillet over medium-high heat, lightly coat the bottom with oil and sauté the mushrooms until soft. Stir in the garlic and season to taste with salt and pepper. Sauté for about 5 to 6 minutes while stirring occasionally.

3.While sautéing the mushrooms, add the milk, eggs, grated Parmesan in separate mixing bowl and whisk until well combined. Season to taste with salt and pepper and briefly mix to combine. Set aside.

4.Place the spinach evenly on the bottom of the prepared pie dish and place the sautéed mushrooms on top. Add the crumbled feta cheese evenly on top of the mushrooms and pour in the egg mixture. Add the shredded Mozzarella cheese evenly over the egg mixture, place it on a baking sheet and bake it in the oven for about 40 to 45 minutes or until the center is set and cooked through.

5.Remove from the oven, transfer on a wire rack and let it rest for about 5 minutes before serving. Slice into 6 equal portions and serve immediately.

6.Spray a pie dish with non-stick spray. Squeeze the rest of the water out of the spinach and spread it out on the bottom of the pie dish. Next add the cooked mushrooms and crumbled feta.

# Baked Broccoli And Marinated Hemp Fu

Preparation time: 20 minutes

Cooking time: 40 to 45 minutes

Serves: 4 to 6

Ingredients:

• 1 block firm hemp or soy tofu, drained and pressed, cut into 1-inch cubes

• 1 red sweet pepper, quartered

• 1 cup of detached broccoli florets

• 1 cup of detached cauliflower florets


• Real salt and black pepper, to taste

For the Marinade:

• ¼ cup raw coconut aminos or namu shoyu

• 1 medium lemon, juiced

• 1 ½ tablespoons of agave nectar

• 1 tablespoon of extra-virgin olive oil

• 1 teaspoon of minced garlic

• 1 small shallot minced

• 1-inch piece of fresh ginger root, minced or grated


• 1 teaspoon of Italian seasoning mix

**Directions:**


1.Mix together all marinade ingredients in a large bowl, add in the tofu and gently toss to evenly coat with the marinade. Cover bowl and chill for at least 1 hour to marinate the tofu.

170

2.Preheat the oven to 375ºF and line two rimmed baking sheets with foil. Set aside.

3.When the tofu is ready, drain and transfer into the prepared baking sheet. Add the vegetables into the marinade mixture and gently toss to coat evenly. Transfer into the prepared baking sheet and bake for 15 minutes in the oven. Turn tofu and vegetables and bake further for about 15 to 20 minutes. Remove from the oven when the tofu is thoroughly cooked and the vegetables are tender.

4.Portion the vegetables into individual serving plates, top with tofu and serve immediately.

# White Bean Soup With Kale And Wild Rice

Preparation time: 10 minutes

Cooking time: 50 to 60 minutes

Serves: 4 to 6

Ingredients:

- 4 cups of homemade vegetable stock or broth
- 1 tablespoon of grass fed ghee or olive oil
- 1 ½ cups of soaked navy beans or canned
- 1 ½ cups wild rice, rinsed and drained
- 1 cup of tomato concasse
- 1 cup diced white onion
- 2 teaspoons of minced garlic
- 2 teaspoons of mixed Italian herbs
- Real salt and black pepper, to taste
- ½ cup coconut cream
- 2 tablespoons of coconut flour
- 1 cup packed fresh kale leaves, roughly chopped

- 1 stem of green onions, chopped

**Directions:**

1.In a large heavy bottomed stock pot, apply medium-high heat and add the ghee or oil. Sauté the onion, garlic and tomato for about 3 to 4 minutes, or until soft and fragrant.

2.Add in the stock, beans, rice and Italian herbs, cover the pot and cook until it reaches to a boil. Reduce to low heat, briefly stir the ingredients and cover the pot. Simmer for about 40 to 50 minutes or until the rice and beans are soft and cooked through.

3.While simmering the soup, dissolve the flour in a bowl with ¼ cup stock and set aside.

4.When the soup is ready, pour in the coconut cream and flour mixture and season to taste with salt and black pepper. Add in the kale and cook until lightly wilted. Remove from heat and adjust seasoning if desired.

5.Portion into individual serving bowls, top with green onions and serve warm.

# Broccoli And Fava Bean Salad

Preparation time: 10 minutes

Cooking time: 10 minutes

Serves: 4

Ingredients:

- 2 cups of boiled fava beans
- 1 cup of boiled green peas
- 2 cups of detached broccoli florets, blanched
- 1 medium red sweet pepper, seeded and sliced into thin strips
- 1 large shallot, thinly sliced
- ½ teaspoon mixed Italian herbs
- Real salt and black pepper, to taste
- 1 teaspoon of toasted sesame seeds, for serving

- 1 teaspoon of chopped fresh parsley, for serving

For the Salad Dressing:

- 1 organic lemon, juiced
- ¼ cup of tahini sauce
- 1 teaspoon of agave nectar

- 1 teaspoon of crushed red pepper flakes

**Directions:**

1.Blanch the broccoli in a pot with boiling water for about 1 to 2 minutes. Remove form pot, transfer to a bowl with ice bath to stop further cooking. Drain, transfer to a large bowl and set aside.

2.In a small mixing bowl, add all salad dressing ingredients and stir until well combined. Set aside.

3.In the large bowl with the broccoli, add in the fava beans, green peas, sweet pepper, shallots and Italian herbs. Season to taste with salt and pepper and pour in the salad dressing.

4.Gently toss to evenly coat the vegetables with the dressing mixture and portion into individual serving bowls.

5.Top with sesame seeds and parsley, chill before serving or serve immediately

# Grilled Vegetables And Hemp Tofu

Preparation time: 15 minutes

Cooking time: 10 to 15 minutes

Serves: 4 to 6

Ingredients:

• 8 ounces pressed and drained Hemp or soy tofu, cut into 4 equal portions
• 1 medium white onions, quartered
• 1 sweet potato, quartered

• 1 large sweet pepper, quartered

For the Marinade:

• 1 tablespoon of tomato paste
• 1 tablespoon of raw coconut aminos
• 1 teaspoon extra-virgin olive oil
• 1 teaspoon liquid stevia or 1 tablespoon agave nectar
• 1 tablespoon prepared mustard
• ½ teaspoon garlic powder

• Salt and black pepper, to taste

**Directions:**

1.Mix all ingredients for the marinade and stir until well combined. Add the Hemp Fu and toss to evenly coat with the marinade mixture. Let it stand for at least 1 hour before grilling and soak two wooden skewers in water.

2.While marinating the Hemp tofu, preheat grill to high and lightly brush the grids with oil.

3.After marinating the Hemp tofu, drain skewers and wipe with paper towels.

4.Thread the onion, a slice of Hemp tofu, a quarter of sweet potato, and a slice of sweet pepper. Repeat the order of threading with the remaining ingredients.

5.Reduce the grill heat to medium and grill the vegetables and Hemp tofu for about 8 to 10 minutes while turning occasionally to cook evenly on all sides.

6.While grilling, regularly brush with remaining marinade and discard the skewers from the grilled Hemp tofu.

7.Let it rest for about 5 minutes before serving placed in a serving platter.

# Quinoa -Fava Green Salad With Avocado Sauce

Preparation time: 15 minutes

Cooking time: N/A minutes

Serves: 4 to 6

Ingredients:

For the salad:

- 2 cups of precooked quinoa
- 2 cup of shelled fresh fava beans
- 1 medium head of lettuce, cored and coarsely chopped
- 1 tablespoon of flax oil
- 2 tablespoons of toasted almonds, chopped

- Real salt and black pepper, to taste

For the Avocado Sauce:

- 1 large ripe avocado, pitted and diced
- 2 organic limes, juiced
- 2 to 3 teaspoons of flax or olive oil
- 1 green jalapeño pepper, seeded and chopped
- 2 tablespoons of minced fresh cilantro leaves
- ½ teaspoon of Italian seasoning mix

- ½ teaspoon coriander powder

**Directions:**

1.Add all sauce ingredients in food processor or high blender and pulse until thick and smooth. Transfer into a small bowl and set aside.

2.In a separate large bowl, add all salad ingredients and season to taste with salt and pepper.

3.Serve salad with avocado sauce on a separate sauce bowl.

# Vegetable Pasta Dinner Recipes
## Carrot Noodles With Spicy Peanut Sauce

Preparation time: 10 minutes

Cooking time: 15 minutes

Serves: 6

Ingredients:

- 1 pound carrots, peeled and spiralized
- 1 tablespoon of toasted sesame oil
- Real salt and black pepper, to taste

- ½ teaspoon of crushed red pepper flakes

For the Sauce:

- 1 tablespoon of extra virgin olive oil
- ½ teaspoon garlic powder
- 1 stem of green onions, chopped
- 1-inch piece of fresh ginger root, minced
- 2 tablespoons of tahini sauce
- ½ cup of unsweetened creamy peanut butter
- 1 teaspoon Sriracha sauce
- ¼ cup raw coconut aminos or namu shoyu
- 2 tablespoons of apple cider vinegar

- 1 tablespoon agave nectar

**Directions:**

1.With a vegetable spiralizer or mandolin, form the carrots into long and thin noodles and transfer into a large bowl.

2.In a small nonstick skillet, apply medium-high heat and add the olive oil. One the oil is hot, sauté the shallot and garlic for about

1 to 2 minutes or until soft and fragrant. Stir in the green onions and ginger, sauté for 2 minutes while stirring regularly until lightly brown and aromatic. Add in the remaining sauce ingredients and bring to a boil. Reduce to low heat and simmer until thick and smooth, while stirring constantly. Remove from heat and set aside to cool.

3.In a separate large skillet, apply medium-high heat add the sesame oil. Add the carrot noodles and stir fry for about 1 to 2 minutes, or lightly brown and crisp. Season to taste with salt and black pepper, remove from heat and transfer into a large serving bowl.

4.Add in the peanut sauce and gently toss to evenly coat the carrot noodles with the sauce. Portion in individual serving salad bowls, top with red pepper flakes and serve immediately.

# Butternut Squash Noodles With Bean Bolognese

Preparation time: 15 minutes

Cooking time: 30 minutes

Serves: 4 to 6

Ingredients:

- 1 pound butternut squash, spiralized
- 1 tablespoon of minced fresh parsley leaves

- ½ cup freshly grated fat free Parmesan cheese

For the Bean Bolognese Sauce:

- 2 tablespoons extra-virgin olive oil
- ½ cup of minced white onion
- ½ cup of minced carrot
- 1 medium stalk of celery, finely chopped
- ½ teaspoon of real salt
- ¼ teaspoon of ground black pepper
- 2 to 3 teaspoons of minced garlic
- 1 ½ cups of canned white beans, rinsed and drained
- 1 teaspoon mixed Italian herbs
- 1 dried laurel or bay leaf
- 2 tablespoons of dry sherry or rice wine
- ¼ cup vegetable stock

- 2 cups of tomato concasse or diced and seeded

**Directions:**

1.Spiralize the butternut squash and blanch for about 1 to 2 minutes in a large pot with boiling water. Remove from the pot, transfer into a large bowl with ice bath to stop further cooking and drain completely. Transfer into a bowl and set aside.

2.In a medium skillet or pan, apply with medium heat and add the oil. Sauté the onions, carrots and celery for about 8 to 10 minutes and season to taste with salt and black pepper. Add in the remaining sauce ingredients and cook until it reaches to a boil. Reduce to low heat and simmer for about 15 to 20 minutes, or until the sauce has thickened and the beans are cooked through. Remove from heat, discard bay leaf and set aside to cool completely.

3.Portion the squash noodles into individual serving bowls and top with sauce. Garnish with grated Parmesan and parsley and serve immediately.

# Cucumber Noodles In Creamy Coconut Mushroom Sauce

Preparation time: 15 minutes

Cooking time: 20 minutes

Serves: 4

Ingredients:

- 2 large cucumbers, spiralized
- 1 tablespoon of olive oil
- 2 tablespoons of minced fresh parsley

- Real salt and black pepper, to taste

For the Sauce:

- ¼ cup of grass fed or vegan butter
- 2 cups of sliced fresh Cremini or button mushrooms
- 2 teaspoons of minced garlic
- 2 tablespoons of coconut flour
- 1 teaspoon mixed Italian herbs
- 1 cup of unsweetened almond or coconut milk

- ½ cup of fresh or unsweetened coconut cream

**Directions:**

1.With a vegetable spiralizer or mandolin, form the cucumbers into long and thick noodles and sprinkle with ¼ teaspoon of salt. Transfer into a colander or strainer and let it stand for about 10 to 15 minutes to drain excess water.

2.Prepare mushroom sauce while waiting for the cucumbers to be done. Add 2 tablespoons of butter in a medium skillet and apply with medium-high heat. Add a teaspoon of minced garlic and sauté for about 1 to 2 minutes, or until lightly golden and fragrant. Stir in the mushrooms, sauté for 6 to 8 minutes while stirring occasionally until soft and tender. Remove from heat, transfer to a plate and set aside.

3.In the same skillet over medium heat, melt the remaining butter and sauté the remaining garlic until soft and fragrant. Sprinkle with flour and Italian herbs and cook until lightly browned and aromatic.

4.Gradually pour in the milk while stirring constantly until the mixture is smooth and well incorporated. Cook until it reaches to a boil while whisking regularly and add the cream. Reduce to low heat, season to taste with salt and pepper and simmer until smooth and thick. Remove from heat and set aside to cool completely.

5.When the cucumbers are ready, toss in the olive oil and parsley and season to taste with salt and pepper. Pour in the sauce and gently toss to evenly coat the cucumber noodles with the sauce mixture.

6.Portion into individual serving bowls and serve immediately with extra parsley on top, if desired.

# Spinach Zucchini Lasagna With Caramelized Onions

Preparation time: 15 minutes

Cooking time: 45 to 60 minutes

Serves: 4 to 6

Ingredients:

- 2 large zucchini, peeled and cut into 4 or 6 lengthwise slices
- Salt and ground black pepper, to taste
- ¼ cup of chopped almonds or walnuts, for the toppings

- ¼ cup finely chopped fresh basil, for the toppings

For the Caramelized Onion Mixture:

- 2 tablespoons of grass fed ghee or extra virgin olive oil
- 2 medium white onions, halved and thinly sliced
- 1 cup diced raw Portabello mushroom caps

- ¼ cup of dry red wine

For the Spinach Filling:

- 2 cups of loosely packed baby spinach
- 1 teaspoon of mixed Italian herbs
- 1 cup of ricotta cheese
- ½ cup tomato puree
- ½ cup chopped fresh basil

- ½ teaspoon salt

For the Sauce and Toppings:

- ¾ cup of almond milk

• ½ cup of soft goat's cheese

**Directions:**

1.With a mandolin or vegetable spiralizer, slice the zucchini into long thin strips and sprinkle with ¼ teaspoon of salt. Gently toss to evenly distribute the salt and place it on a colander to drain excess water from the zucchini.

2.In a large nonstick skillet or pan, apply medium-low heat and add 1 tablespoon of oil. Add in the onions and cook for about 15 to 20 minutes while stirring occasionally until the soft and caramelized. Add in the remaining oil and stir in the mushrooms. Cook further for about 5 to 6 minutes, or until the mushrooms are soft and tender. Pour in the wine and cook until it reaches to a boil while scraping the browned bits on the bottom of the skillet. Season to taste with salt and black pepper, remove skillet from heat and set aside.

3.In a food processor or high speed blender, combine together all filling ingredients and pulse until thick and smooth. Transfer to a bowl, cover and set aside.

4.Preheat the oven to 375°F and lightly grease a baking dish with oil, set aside.

5.Prepare the sauce while preheating the oven. In a medium saucepan over medium heat, pour in the milk and cook until it reaches to a simmer. Add in the cheese and cook for about 3 to 5 minutes while stirring constantly until the cheese is fully melted. Remove from heat and set aside.

6.In the prepared baking dish, add about ¼ cup milk-cheese mixture and spread evenly on the bottom with spatula. Layer half of the sliced zucchini and top with half of the spinach filling mixture. Spread the spinach filling evenly on top and a layer of half the caramelized onion mixture.

7.Start the second layer with the remaining sliced zucchini. Cover with the remaining spinach filling and spread the rest of the caramelized onion mixture on top. Pour in the remaining milk-cheese sauce and spread evenly on top. Sprinkle with chopped nuts and parsley and bake it in the oven for about 25 to 30 minutes.

8.Remove from the oven, transfer to a wire rack and let it rest for about 10 minutes before serving.

# Conclusion

Since you have reached this point in the book, you should now have an idea of the foods you can enjoy on your 21-Day Sugar Detox Diet. It is important to remember that the detox diet is not about depriving your body of carbohydrates and sugars. Rather, it is about replacing carb- and sugar-laden foods with more wholesome foods for improved energy and better overall health.

The next logical step is to make a shopping list and start planning! Come up with a meal list and then head to the grocery store. If you plan ahead, you may even be able to get all your foods ready in a single day out of the week. Then, you can throw together most of your meals in half an hour or less.

CPSIA information can be obtained
at www.ICGtesting.com
Printed in the USA
BVHW032255261022
650444BV00010B/84

9 781990 169878